How To Overcome STRESS Naturally

Take Control of Your Mental & Emotional Life...

Foreword by
His Holiness
The Dalai Lama

TRACEY STRANGER

DISCLAIMER

The information in this book is for educational purposes only and is not intended to replace the advice of physicians or health care practitioners. It is also not intended to diagnose or prescribe treatment for any illness or disorder. Anyone already undergoing physician-prescribed therapy should seek the advice of his or her doctor before reducing their dosage or stopping such treatment.

FIRST EDITION 2009

National Library of Australia
Cataloguing-in-Publication entry:

Stranger, Tracey, 1958-
How to overcome stress naturally / Tracey Stranger.

1st ed.
ISBN: 978-1-925370-28-7 ebook
ISBN: 978-1-921630-07-1 p/b

1. Stress management 2. Depression, Mental--Alternative treatment

A catalogue record for this book is available from the National Library of Australia

NATIONAL LIBRARY OF AUSTRALIA

Published by Global Publishing Group
PO Box 258, Banyo Qld 4014
Email. admin@GlobalPublishingGroup.com.au

For Further information about orders:
Phone: +61 7 3267 0747

Praise For
How To Overcome Stress Naturally

*"**Don't Worry, Be Happy!** This book shows you how to begin your personal journey to change your life, your mindset, your eating habits and your friends – well maybe not all of them! For all of us, something needs changing and this book contains real gems to help you achieve your own amazing potential."*

John Kumm, Bestselling Author
Get Packing - Your Ultimate Travel Guide

"The Dalai Lama says Without Inner Peace, How can we Make Real Peace. With these natural and practical solutions you have a day-to-day plan to help you reach you own inner peace. Take this opportunity – compelling reading."

Verena Cunningham, Author of "The Joy of Conscious Living" and Director of "The Australian Institute of Self Development"

"There are no secrets. You have all the answers. The "How To" and "Then What" is explained step-by-step giving you an abundance of choices to take control of your health and your wealth today."

Andrew Carter, Author, Speaker, Coach and Entrepreneur

"This book will dramatically improve your health and your wealth in a truly down to earth way and easy to implement on a day-to-day basis."

Dr. Gordon Ku, Author of "Dr. House's Prescription To Escape The 9 To 5"

"This is a very timely and succinct book for our current time of great change. With stress and depression so close for so many; Tracey offers a holistic approach including Ayurvedic, Integrative, Nutritional and Environmental methods. This gives people a real power of choice with easy to follow actions. In a world where so many turn first to drugs, Tracey offers a breath of fresh air by providing this natural self-help way forward for everyday stress BEFORE it leads to depression."

Steven Broadbent
Author of Your Sacred Path – from the Dancer to the Dance and the Secret Within You

"Say no to financial stress. Say yes to change. The first step is to accept it's time to change. The world is changing. This book can help you change providing day-to-day guidance and inspirational personal stories. You too can change – don't wait, start to take control now. "

Nicholas de Castella, Director, Institute of Heart Intelligence.

How To Overcome Overcome STRESS Naturally

I live in hope that everyone's spirit can be uplifted so we can all live a positive, peaceful, harmonious life together and enjoy this magnificent planet called Earth.

Tracey Stranger

Acknowledgements

I want to thank my Mum and Dad for who they are and always supporting my sister and I to do what made us happy, whatever our crazy adventures were. I feel blessed to know they were always there for me.

My inspiration for this book came from a close friend who was struggling with depression, as I could see the heartache and despair that affected the whole family. Her mother said to me, "Why don't you write a book on Mental Health? It is so misunderstood by so many people." I thank you for your suggestion for such an important subject.

Within the next 3 days I heard from several close friends who had friends with severe depression, and there had also been 2 suicides. I was experiencing, first hand, that everyone knows someone with depression. I also had friends tell me of their experiences with depression many years ago. Mental health is a major health problem worldwide.

I thank my friends who walk the same path – they know who they are. You are my continual inspiration.

I want to thank the many teachers I have met on my journey that add to the richness of my understanding, never-ending desire to learn and deepen my love and compassion for our fellow human beings, animals and all that is.

I sincerely thank all the contributors to this book with the jewels of knowledge, wisdom, passion and desire to help others by sharing as they have. You truly touched my heart with your sincerity, honesty and openness that I am sure will touch all who read this book.

A very special thank you to Darren Stephens at Global Publishing Group for the invaluable guidance, support and trust in my ability to transform my passion and desire into this book that will help so many.

Thank you the reader, for having this book in your hands to Help You Overcome Stress Naturally, as simple as ABC. When you understand, you can make meaningful choices. As human beings we all have a choice.

Contents

ENCOURAGING STORIES

Foreword

I believe that the purpose of life is to be happy. From the moment of birth, every human being wants happiness and does not want suffering. From the very core of our being, we simply desire contentment.

It is possible to divide every kind of happiness and suffering into two main categories: mental and physical. Of the two, it is the mind that exerts the greatest influence on most of us. Unless we are either gravely ill or deprived of basic necessities, our physical condition plays a secondary role in life. If the body is content, we virtually ignore it. The mind, however, registers every event, no matter how small. Hence, we should devote our most serious efforts to bringing about mental peace.

From my own limited experience, I have found that the greatest degree of inner tranquillity comes from the development of love and compassion.

The more we care for the happiness of others, the greater our own sense of well-being becomes. Cultivating a close, warm-hearted feeling for others automatically puts the mind at ease. This helps remove whatever fears or insecurities we may have and gives us the strength to cope with any obstacles we encounter. It is the ultimate source of success in life.

As long as we live in this world, we are bound to encounter problems. If, at such times, we lose hope and become discouraged, we diminish our ability to face difficulties. If, on the other hand, we remember that it is not just ourselves but everyone who has to undergo suffering. This more realistic perspective will increase our determination and capacity to overcome troubles. Indeed, with this attitude, each new obstacle can be seen as yet another valuable opportunity to improve our mind!

Thus, we can strive gradually to become more compassionate, that is we can develop both genuine sympathy for others suffering and the will to help remove their pain. As a result, our own serenity and inner strength will increase.

Ultimately, the reason why love and compassion bring the greatest happiness is simply that our nature cherishes them above all else. The need for love lies at the very foundation of human existence. It results from the profound interdependence we all share with one another. However capable and skilful an individual may be, left alone, he or she will not survive. However vigorous and independent one may feel during the most prosperous periods of life, when one is sick, very young or very old, one must depend on the support of others.

We have to consider what we human beings really are. We are not like machine-made objects. If we are merely mechanical entities, then machines themselves could alleviate all of our sufferings and fulfil our needs.

However, since we are not solely material creatures, it is a mistake to place all our hopes for happiness on external development alone. Instead, we should consider our origins and nature to discover what we require.

Compassion contributes to good physical health as well. According to my personal experience, mental stability and physical well-being are directly related. Without question, anger and agitation make us more susceptible to illness. On the other hand, if the mind is tranquil and occupied with positive thoughts, the body will not easily fall prey to disease.

We need to make a concerted effort to develop compassion; we must use all the events of our daily life to transform our thoughts and behaviour. True compassion is not just an emotional response but a firm commitment founded on reason. Therefore, a truly compassionate attitude towards others does not change even if they behave negatively.

Of course, developing this kind of compassion is not at all easy! Let me emphasize that it is within your power, given patience and time, to develop this kind of compassion. Compassion is by nature gentle, peaceful and soft, but it is very powerful.

Though sometimes people laugh when I say it, I myself always want more friends. I love smiles. Because of this I have the problem of knowing how to make more friends and how to get more smiles, in particular, genuine smiles. For there are many kinds of smile, such as sarcastic, artificial or diplomatic smiles. Many smiles produce no feeling of satisfaction, and sometimes they can even create suspicion or fear, can't they? But a genuine smile really gives us a feeling of freshness and is, I believe, unique to human beings. If these are the smiles we want, then we ourselves must create the reasons for them to appear.

Individual happiness can contribute in a profound and effective way to the overall improvement of our entire human community. Because we all share an identical need for love, it is possible to feel that anybody we meet, in whatever circumstances, is a brother or sister. No matter how new the face or how different the dress and behaviour, there is no significant division between us and other people.

If you have a sincere and open heart, you naturally feel self-worth and confidence, and there is no need to be fearful of others. I believe that at every level of society - familial, tribal, national and international - the key to a happier and more successful world is the growth of compassion. We do not need to become religious, nor do we need to believe in an ideology. All that is necessary is for each of us to develop our good human qualities.

In this book the author brings the professional expertise from western medicine, Ayurvedic Medicine, Integrative Western & Complementary Medicine and Nutrition Medicine together to provide understanding and choices. The personal stories with heartfelt pain and recovery, practical daily activities and meditations and a personalised Day-To-Day Plan on How to Overcome Stress Naturally, are aimed to help prevent the spiral into Depression and lift your spirit.

In today's economic and world climate everyday moods of frustration, anger, hopelessness, anxiety and fear, it is ever more important to truly understand the power of the Mind and cultivate love and compassion daily.

Tenzin Gyatso; The Fourteenth Dalai Lama of Tibet

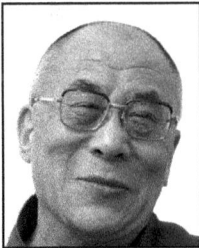

Introduction

Stressed? Stress is necessary for normal function of the body. A signal of stress at a cellular level triggers a chain reaction for the body to find its homeostatic balance again. The body has an incredible ability to bring itself back to balance. So much so we don't think about it, it happens every day.

We only begin to notice when we start to feel uncomfortable. If we are uncomfortable, or stressed, for too long, we often become dis-eased. That's how we can progress from stress to depression, which is an illness or dis-ease.

The aim of this book is to Overcome Stress Naturally before the downward cycle of depression begins.
What are the signs of stress? We each have our own level of tolerance. What is "stressful" for one, is not "stressful" for another, on a physical, emotional and mental level.

The key is to get to the heart of the matter for you. This book is the ABC of Overcoming Stress Naturally.
Firstly, Accept the situation and Acknowledge you are "stressed". Now Breathe; stop still for a moment and take a Deep Breath. Oxygen is vital at a cellular level and it also helps us to relax and calm down. Then Change your Attitude, Change your Response, Change your Thoughts, Change Something!

Stress is a signal that it's time to change something. It is your task to restore balance on all levels.
Take control of your mental and emotional wellbeing. Step by Step it can be done, naturally.
The human body is an incredible creation and we can heal ourselves naturally when we know how.
It is my intention that the information and resources in this book help you to understand the choices you have, and where you can go for help to find your personal unique journey to inner balance and peace, naturally.
Live the life that is true to you, with love in your heart for yourself and for all those around you.

"Without Inner Peace, How can we Make Real Peace?"
The Dalai Lama.

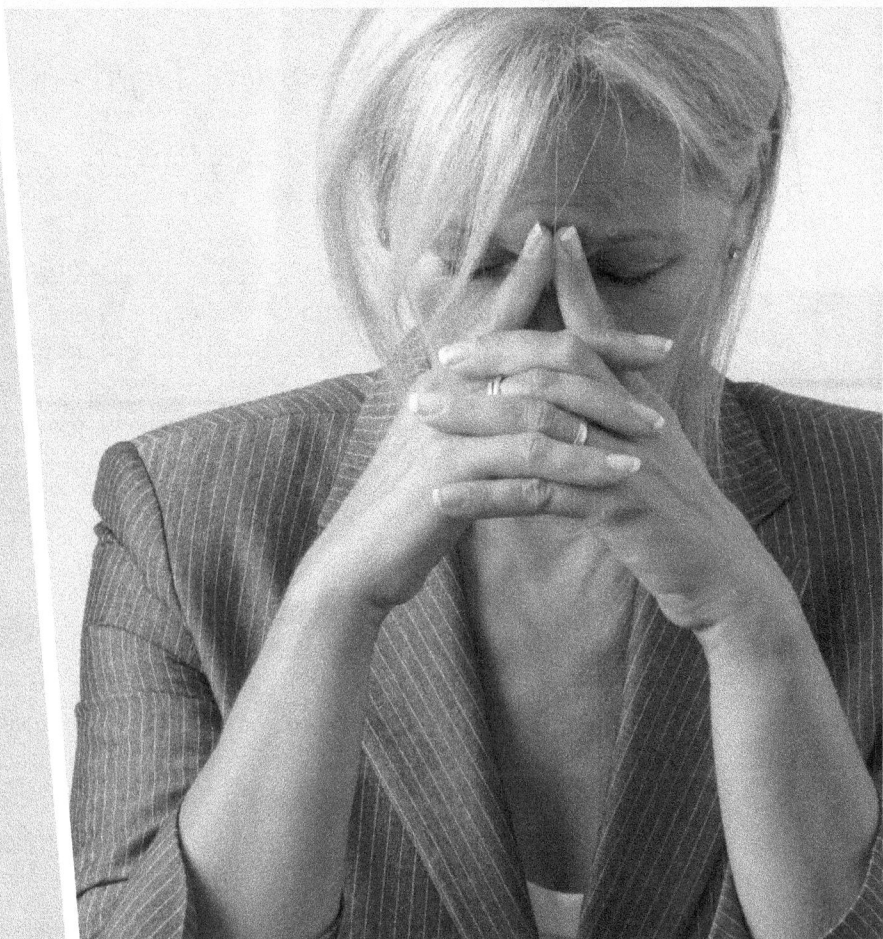

Chapter 1:

Stress, Mood Disorders, Depression

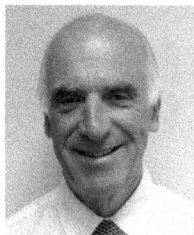

Chapter 1:

Stress, Mood Disorders, Depression

Prof Gordon Parker: Executive Director:
Black Dog Institute, NSW

Widespread stress prevailed in the land. Some scientists decided to define stress which can lead to depression and research this to understand patterns of behaviour and causes. It is a growing trend with the development of humanity, technology, medicine, agriculture. Whilst the rewards are many, the stress level seems to grow. No-one escapes. It is a roller coaster effect.

Like a deck of cards, it only takes one person to be stressed and the effect seems to ripple through to the many. Alternatively, if one person can hold themselves in Balance & Love, it also seems to have a ripple effect to the many. The key is Compassion.

1 in 5 Australians will experience some form of mental illness each year.[1]

Mental illness affects young people; at least 1/3 of young people have had an episode of mental illness by the age of 25 years.[2]

Edgar Cayce was decades ahead of modern medical research when he gave graphic descriptions of nervous system pathology in cases of depression. Instead of relying heavily on medication to alter the chemical imbalance in the nervous system, he would usually recommend more natural methods. These "holistic" therapies would help the body to be its own "medicine chest" and thus bring its faulty biochemistry back into a healthy state. "Mind is the builder" is a prominent theme in the readings, and is based upon the inherent association of mental processes with the nervous system.[3]

Chapter 1: *Stress, Mood Disorders, Depression*

Prof Parker, tell us about the Black Dog Institute, who they are, and a bit about what you do?

We did have an earlier organization, which was called the Mood Disorders Unit, which was a clinical research facility for people with a mood disorder. Our definition of mood disorder means 'somebody with clinical depression' and 'people with a bi-polar disorder'; so there are two differing mood conditions that we focus on. In 2002, we formed the Black Dog Institute to build on the successes of the Mood Disorders Unit and to expand it, so that we might help many more people.

As a consequence of receiving funding from the New South Wales government, we would focus on providing support, services and information to people in New South Wales; but that has expanded.

The Black Dog Institute model essentially involves four key components—and I really don't know of any other institute in Australia that's got four components.

1. We've got clinical services where we have a very strong research component and track record.

2. We run professional education for psychiatrists, psychologists, school counsellors, and for special groups; i.e. large organizations, police and armed forces.

3. We also run educational programs for people in the community; so education is a big component.

4. The final of the four various nodes is that of a community enterprise. We have a walk-in community centre that has a library and we run support groups for people with mood disorders, and for their families.

More importantly, we go out from the Institute via our website, and I'm very proud of the website. We're now running at about 150,000 hits a month, and it is a very rich website for people in the community, with very up-to-date information.

There are fact sheets on the mood disorders; and they're up-to-date in the sense that if you're a woman, and you have a mood disorder, and you're going to have a baby, and you want to know whether certain medications are safe, you can go on and get pretty up-to-date information.

We allow people to take part in screening tests to assess their depression levels and whether they might have a bi-polar disorder. So, we give information; we help people in terms of sub-typing their particular mood disorder; and then we also, via the web, run some educational packages.

Just to give an example, we have an eighty-minute educational program on bi-polar disorder, with ten professionals contributing to that—and of the ten, five have bi-polar disorder themselves.

What I think is equally important is that it's an integrative model, so each of the four nodes informs the other nodes. So if we find out something in our research node, that gets fed through to our clinical management of people; gets through to our professional education; it gets fed through to our community education; it gets fed through on the web.

I think it's been a wonderful organization to be involved with, because we have also contributed a lot to destigmatization of mood disorders in this country. It's a rich model.

I suppose the other component that I'd mention is that we do publish quite a lot of material, and we've put out four books on depression for the general reader: a book called "*Journey Through the Black Dog*", one on bi-polar disorder called "*Mastering Bi-Polar*" and a couple of others.

Chapter 1: *Stress, Mood Disorders, Depression*

The Black Dog Institute's website has various questionnaires linking personality with depression, which are excellent tools for self understanding.

Visit www.blackdoginstitute.org.au

Yes, and there's also a toolkit on the website—we've got that in our General Practitioner Education module- but anyone can go anywhere on our website. The toolkit allows people to download various tools, i.e. on relaxation.

We not only focus on mood disorder, we're moving more and more into positive psychology and well-being. There's a fact sheet on happiness, and there's another fact sheet on positive psychology; so, it's pretty rich.

How would you define the difference between depression, mood disorder and chronic stress?

Let me start with stress, because I think that's the most difficult one to define.

I think that stress is psychological and physiological, and because it straddles both components it is a bit vague in terms of how we seek to define it. It can vary dimensionally. We can come home at the end of the day and say we've had a stressful day, where an objective outsider might say, "Well, that's just trivial."

The model that I have found helpful is one which was really developed by Selye, in the 1930s, and he talks about a general adaptation syndrome.

This means that an individual must have some sort of stimulus, **Basically, there are three stages to this process: alarm, resistance, and exhaustion.** or set of stimuli, that triggers off a stress reaction.

The first stage, alarm, is when the individual is aware that they are in danger—which is usually conscious for us human beings, but can sometimes almost be unconscious. I mean, you could be swimming in the water, and you might see a shadow; and some atavistic, primitive mechanism- "Maybe this is a shark", when it's not a shark- can be sufficient to stimulate that alarm phase.

Basically what happens is the body pours out adrenaline and cortisol, and this prepares the human being for the well known flight or fight response; blood pressure goes up, and heart rate increases, and all of these strategies that are built within us to protects us. That's the first stage.

That can't go on forever, and so there's a second stage, of resistance- this is where the parasympathetic nervous system, as against the sympathetic one, comes into play, and heart rate and breathing rate return to normal.

At this stage, the human being is remaining on alert; they're still prepared for action, but they're beginning to adapt to the stress, psychologically and physically. Nevertheless, that takes its toll, and we're also now aware that the immunological system is brought into play here.

It's basically like traffic lights; you've now gone into the yellow light, and you're not sure whether the light's going to go red or green, or whatever.

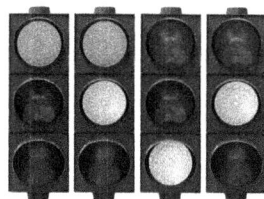

Then there's the third phase of exhaustion. At this stage the stress has gone on for a decent period; it is at a sufficiently severe level to be significant, and the person has exhausted their repertoire. At this stage you start to get psychological problems at a pretty severe level— whether we call them stress, whether we call it anxiety, whether we call it depression, they're all outcomes that can be differentiated from each other.

Also, the individual's bodily function is compromised. The immune system is highly activated, T-cells may be depleted, so people are more likely to get physical illnesses at those times, and also they're feeling much more exhausted. They've gone through that stage of alert alarm, to feeling fatigued and exhausted.

Chapter 1: *Stress, Mood Disorders, Depression*

The time frame is going to be different for everybody, depending on intensity?

Yes, that's right. Some people will only get into the first stage, because the threat may abort, they'll settle down. Some people get to the second stage; some people get to the third stage.

There are going to be some differences in the time length depending on the situation and the individual, but the time differences don't vary quite so much as the severity.

The stress response as I would see it is there for a purpose. That's important to recognise, because if it's there for a purpose that means it's normal. It's there to protect us in terms of an evolutionary mechanism.

Getting to the third phase, as you call it, when the stress has continued on for a period of time and intensity, may it manifest as more severe mood disorders or depression?

The next thing we need to say is: How do we define anxiety? How do we define depression? How do we define grief? They are three common consequences of stress.

To my mind, anxiety is a response of fear; the individual feels insecure, and in extreme versions, they feel as if they're going mad. So if any patient comes into my office and says,"Doctor, I think I'm going mad," I think 'anxiety until proven otherwise'.

Depression is not only feeling depressed, but there's a drop in one's sense of self-esteem or self-worth, and people tend to be fairly self-critical. The only exception, having said all that, is sometimes when somebody has a psychotic depression, and they just feel incredibly physically fatigued, and lacking in energy. If you ask them about their self-esteem, they sometimes don't know what you're talking about, or they'll say that doesn't cut it for me.

Most of the time, using that as a definition of depression, I ask three questions:

> Are you feeling depressed?
> Has there been a drop in your self-esteem / self-worth?
> Are you feeling any more self critical?

These help describe a mood state of depression. And that does not mean clinical depression.

And the third one is grief. Grief is when you've lost something of value, but not your self-esteem. That's really important. It doesn't mean that it's any less severe. Grief can be horribly severe, like the death of a partner or a child; I couldn't think of anything worse. That is not a condition where self-esteem is impacted on. For two-thirds of people, it never happens. For one-third, late in the stage of grief, they can move onto depression. Grief, to my mind, is the loss of something of value that doesn't necessarily involve your self-esteem.

If you take those three definitions, then you're starting the process, logically, of working out whether somebody's likely to have a primary anxiety, a primary depression, or a primary grief.

It doesn't deny that anxious people are often depressed, and depressed people are often anxious, and grief can go onto depression. But to my mind it really is important to make those higher-order, sequencing, first-level diagnoses, because after that, things then start to fall into place.

How do we distinguish depression, as a mood state, from clinical depression?

We did a couple of studies of the general population, a couple of decades ago, and we went up to people in the street, and asked if they have ever experienced those states.

Consider this definition: "You have times when you feel depressed. There's a drop in your self-esteem and self-worth. You feel self-critical. You feel hopeless and helpless. You feel like giving up and you think that people around have given up on you."

Basically, ninety-six percent of people said they have.

I don't doubt that.

Chapter 1: *Stress, Mood Disorders, Depression*

The point of the story is that it's normal to feel depressed.

Then we said, "How often do you feel like that?" In the two studies, one came out as an average of about every two months, and the other one came out about every six weeks. What was different between these states and clinical depression, firstly, was duration. So what I'd suggest is that there is a thing called 'normal depression', or sadness that we all feel when we've been taken down a peg, or we've lost something that we've tied our self-esteem to.

We feel depressed and demoralized. For most human beings there is the capacity for spontaneous remission, after minutes, hours, or days, or when something nice happens. Your football team wins, or somebody calls you up. And that normal depression then just disappears; that sadness disappears.

In clinical depression, we therefore have to say, "Well, how do we get around this problem of defining clinical depression in a way that doesn't set the bar too high or too low?"

I think we have a problem with the definition of the moment. The definition of the moment says that you have to have a depressed mood—and there are various criteria, and to my mind, many of those symptoms are pretty trite.

The risk of the current definition of clinical depression is that it will bring in many people that are just really experiencing normal depression, which is lasting a bit longer and is maybe a bit more severe.

I do think we've had a problem in the last twenty years, where clinical depression has been defined a bit too easily, and has not been well-distinguished from normal mood states.

That then leads to a whole series of predictable problems of people getting treatment when they actually don't necessarily need treatment. They often can benefit from support, wise counselling, and other strategies.

How do you get to the fundamental root cause of the problem?

We don't agree with the dominant model that's around in Australia and overseas, that depression is just a single condition that varies by severity.

We see that as a very simplistic model that leads to a whole series of problems. We would argue that, within the clinical depressive world of conditions, there are a couple of conditions that are absolutely biological; they are strongly genetically underpinned, and they come out when the neuro-circuits in the brain are disrupted. We talk therefore about psychotic depression, melancholic depression and bi-polar disorder.

These are conditions where there is a biological problem going on at the primary level which may have just come on spontaneously, or may have come on with stress, but it's there and it's able to be reasonably diagnosed.

By contrast, we have the range of what we call non-melancholic disorders, which are more a reflection of the individual's personality, and/or the stresses that they're facing. i.e. somebody might have a personality style of being an extreme worrier, and therefore, they're going to worry that they're not meeting people's expectations, that their spouse isn't happy with them, that their employer isn't happy with them, so constantly they're getting depressed as a consequence of their personality style of worrying.

On the other hand, other people may be getting stressed because of a whole series of life events. We call those social factors, as against personality/psychological factors. They can be acute or chronic.

You might get depressed because of a stress where you're demeaned by your boss, and you feel diminished, and you lose your self-esteem; that's an acute stressor. Or you may have had stresses in the past, of being abused, bullied, sexually abused, or having uncaring parenting; and they've made you extremely vulnerable to stressors which echo those.

Chapter 1: *Stress, Mood Disorders, Depression*

Our view is that it is important to recognise the dimensional model; we just merely put those people along a dimension of severity, which is meaningless. It's like saying to a woman with a breast lump, well that's a big lump, or a small lump…and she doesn't want to know that. She wants to know whether it's a cancer or a benign cyst.

Why is it important? Well, it's important for several reasons. It's more logical to say,"Well, given that there may be depressive subtypes caused by biological, psychological, or social factors, let's get the treatment to try to modulate, modify, correct that factor."

If it's a biological depression, the evidence all stacks up that anti-depressant drugs are probably the best of the lot. If it's a psychological based depression, where the personality is causing the problem, then it may be better to try to help that person to adjust their personality, or their response to stressors, than to give them a drug.

Continuing the paradigm, if stress is causing the depression, then the best thing you might do would be to neutralize the stress—if you could wave a magic wand—or do something in a practical sense, or help the person come to terms with the stress—practically, or by empathically listening to them.

The model basically is saying, if your car's got a problem and you go to the mechanic, you want to know what the problem is, and what's the logical thing that the mechanic will do that'll fix it up.

You can only get there if you can concede that there may be differing types of depression—biological, psychological, social—and having your therapy designed to address those key, causal factors.

That's the Black Dog model, which is in contrast with the general view out there, which I despair. This is where people come along and they get told that they've got clinical depression, severe, moderate, or mild, and then what they get is the treatment that reflects the background training or discipline of the practitioner.

If you've got depression type x and you go to a doctor, you'll probably get a drug; go with the same type of depression to a psychologist, you'll probably get cognitive-behavioural therapy; go to a counsellor, you'll probably get counselling.

This is a procrustean model, where the patient is being fitted to the background training of the therapist—as against the rest of medicine, where treatment is based around what's going on.

How do you incorporate Mindfulness at the Black Dog Institute?

At this stage, we're testing it in several ways. Mindfulness has only come to the attention of psychiatrists and psychologists in recent times, which is a bit embarrassing, but that's the reality.

Anecdotally, I'm impressed with mindfulness. So one of the things we decided to do was a formal trial, comparing the most respected type of psychotherapy, as used by psychologists in Australia at the moment, of cognitive-behavioural therapy (CBT), and to compare that to mindfulness-based CBT. We will publish the results in some months' time; that's a very important study.

Maybe I can just give you a couple of hints: it's probably horses for courses. Mindfulness tends to be particularly good for people who have high levels of anxiety and stress and worry. Secondly, we think we can see faster onset of action with mindfulness, because you're doing something immediately to settle down the stress, the perturbation, the worrying.

What is important is, "In what conditions is it most likely to be particularly effective, and in what conditions is it likely to be ineffective or irrelevant?" That's our horses for courses model for everything.

What would you suggest are some simple, practical first steps to be taking on the path to overcome stresses of daily life?

The first thing is to say,
"Are you actually stressed, in a meaningful sense?"
And I think the next question—if you say yes, you are— is to say,
"Is it all negative? Or is some of it positive?"

I think there's a tendency for most people to say stress is all negative, and we should, therefore, change our lives.

Chapter 1: *Stress, Mood Disorders, Depression*

In fact, there are people who like being stressed to some degree. People jump out of airplanes in parachutes, and people drive cars fast, and many people will work at a level where they're actually raising their stress levels—because they feel alive; they feel a buzz.

I think the second question is,
"If you are stressed, then is it satisfying stress?

Does it give you something that makes you feel alive?"
Therefore it may not necessarily be quite so negative.

The next sequence is: if you've decided that, yes, you are stressed, and it's got negative components, then I think there are several ways.

One is that you can internally reflect and say,
"Well, what am I going to do about it?"

One is to get a treatment, which basically says, you're not going to change your life, but you're just going to try and knock the stress level down by some drug or non-drug strategy.

Or, you can say,
"Well, how can I change my life, where I'll preserve what's important, but try to get the stress levels down?"
1. One can do that by internal reflection;
2. If you're lucky enough to have a partner who's empathic, you can discuss it with them, and so build them into the solution;
3. Some people will do it by counselling.

If you decide you're going to do something about the stress, there are two broad options in the sequence.
1. **You can say, "I will change my day-to-day procedures." OR**
2. **"I will actually change my job," OR something else like that.**

I actually, personally, believe that for many of us, if we're lucky enough, there may be an ecological niche in our life where we can actually find the job we want, and the home life that we want—without necessarily changing ourselves. For others, that's exactly the wrong way to go; and we need to actually change ourselves.

There are many patients that I will see who might come along; and I think they're stressed merely because they're just in the wrong job; and I will suggest to them, well why don't you try this or that or whatever. They may end up working exactly as many long hours, but they may say, "But it's different. It feels very different to me. I feel there's something about it; it's not just a job, it's a career; it's rewarding." And, therefore, you've effectively addressed their stress levels.

For some people, of course, then you need to, obviously, pursue actual treatments or management strategies. And that becomes horses for courses.

I basically give people the options and say,

"What do you think you'd like to try first?"

And it's quite amazing the variation that I get reported back to me. Some will swear for exercise, and some will swear for meditation.

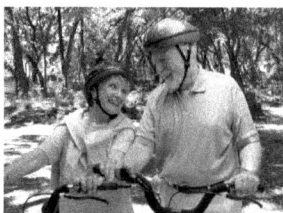

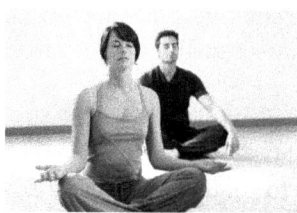

We report our journeys with the Black Dog; we had 650 people write down how they've managed depression. The variety of responses was amazing. Again, meditation and exercise came up very strongly. There are other quixotic ones, like don't listen to talk-back radio. Plus...

**Cut out the negativity in your life;
Just don't allow any people that you associate with to be negative.
Appreciate the positives.**

It is very individual; as we inch our way towards Bethlehem, we need to respect that there are many pathways that can get us there.

There's another aspect here and that is we basically won't change unless we're in a crisis.

Chapter 1: *Stress, Mood Disorders, Depression*

The Chinese symbol for crisis is also the symbol for opportunity to change.

I think as humans, as sentient human beings, we're not just animals who get stressed and avoid the stressor. As human beings, we should be saying, "Ah, isn't that interesting? There's a message. Now, what am I going to do with that message?" Reflect on the fact that we are most likely to commit ourselves to change, and to start the process of change, only when we're stressed.

What inspires you at the start of each day?

I've been very blessed. I did medicine, and I thought I'd be a surgeon. I trained for a while as a surgeon, then I realised I wasn't going to be a very good surgeon. I drifted in medical journalism, and took up psychiatry—and within a few weeks I was just like a pig in mud. I just found it wonderful, and I have retained that sense of enthusiasm for being a psychiatrist. So I wake up each day, if I'm going off to work, and I know it's going to be an interesting day.

I'm lucky enough to have a mix of administration where I feel that I'm building something, seeing good people come along, and having their careers developed.

I've got the clinical contact, and I see quite a lot of people as patients. Not a week goes by that I am not inspired by the way in which people handle stresses, and I learn, every week, something.

Then there's the research. I've always enjoyed the process of creativity.

Outside of work, what inspires me, what gets me going?…Well, it's other things. I was a professional writer for a long period of time, and now I've got a play that's being read in New York in May this year, and that's wonderful. And if my golf handicap comes down, that's wonderful. So it's the richness of life, I guess.

You have a writing competition at the Black Dog Institute.

Yes, we do; every year. And that's very inspiring because, after more than thirty years as a psychiatrist, most of my education has come from books by experts telling me and others what we should do for patients—which is somewhat top-down.

When we have the writing competition, we have people telling us things about what's worked for them—and that's bottom-up information. That's coming from people who've done the hard yards. And there's often a huge disjunction between the two worlds. So the textbooks might say for depression, "Prescribe anti-depressants."

But when you listen to people who've had serious depression and say what works, they take the anti-depressants as a given, but they then say, after that: it was exercise; it was doing this and that, and whatever.

The writing competitions are giving us information from the people who have done the hard yards, who are intelligent, who are prepared to write an essay and put into words—often wonderfully humorous, but often also incredibly profound—information that really does inform us. And we are fools, as professionals, if we just listen to our own professional colleagues, and we don't learn from the people that have had the conditions.

ABC MINDFULNESS FOR TODAY

1. Reflect on your life. Create a quiet moment and review where your greatest negative stress is.

2. ABC - Accept the situation, Breathe Deeply, Change your perspective.
   How can I look at this situation differently?
   What is a positive solution to this situation?
   How can I resolve this discomfort, this stress? Be Creative!

3. ABC – Action, Believe in Yourself, Change your thinking, beliefs, attitude.
   Action – remove yourself from the stressful situation.
   Action – go for a walk, get some fresh air, physically move.
   Action – go to a gym class, aerobics, walk to the corner store.
   Breathe – Remember to Breathe Deeply & Believe in yourself.
   Change your mind. You do have a choice. Change your thinking for a win-win.

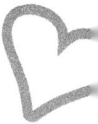

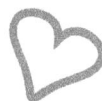

SIMPLE DAILY CONTEMPLATION / MEDITATION

At the START of your day AND at the END of your day... take a few quite minutes for YOU.
BE KIND TO YOURSELF.

Sit comfortably, spine straight, feet and legs uncrossed.
Close your eyes, take a DEEP BREATH IN
As you exhale LET GO of the day, LET GO of all thoughts,
LET GO of all emotions.
Take another DEEP BREATH IN, focus only on your breathing.
As you exhale LET GO even further, LET GO and RELAX,
LET GO of everything.
Take another DEEP BREATH IN, focus only on the breath.
Exhale, focus only on the breath.
Open your eyes.

THAT IS 3 DEEP BREATHS that takes only a minute EVERY DAY.

Notice how you feel.
Do you feel calmer?
Do you feel more relaxed?
Do you feel you are able to make clearer decisions?

**STRIVE TO BUILD THIS UP TO 10 MINUTES EACH DAY.
IT'S A GREAT WAY TO BEGIN EVERY DAY!**

1. Mental Health and Wellbeing: Profile of Adults, Australia 1997, Australian Bureau of Statistics, 1998
2. Making Sense of Orygen Youth Health – www.orygen.org.au
3. www.edgarcayce.org/health/database/health_resources/depression.asp

"I don't think of all the misery but of the beauty that still remains."
Anne Frank.

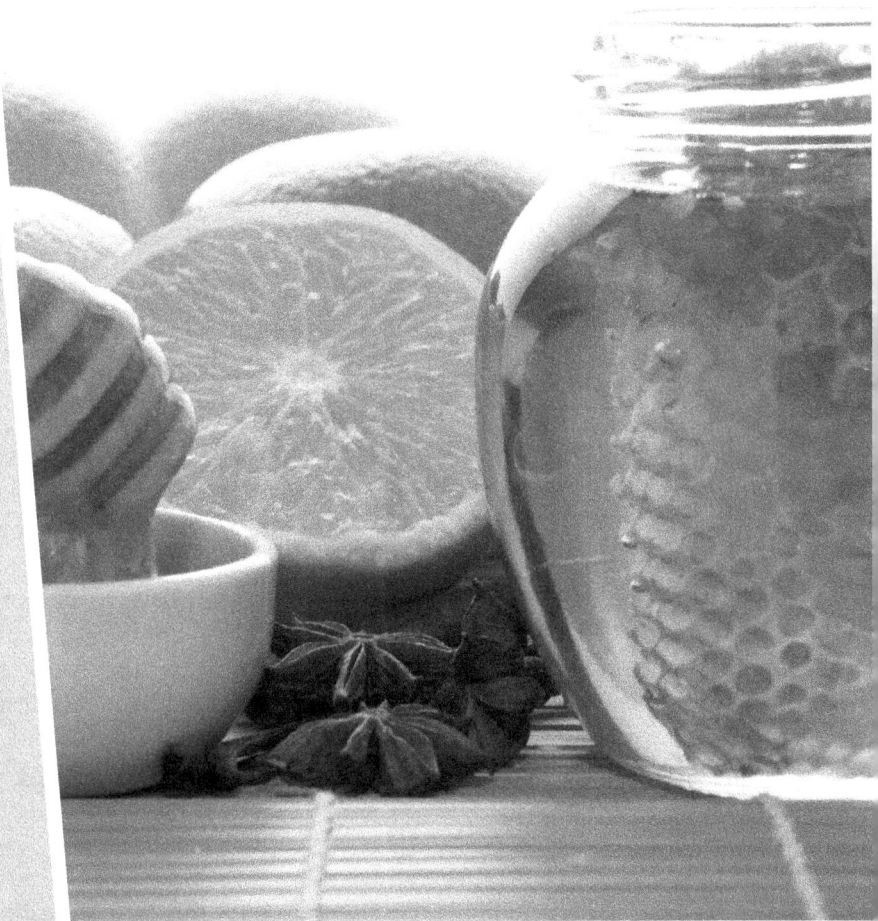

Chapter 2:

Introducing Integrative Medicine –

The Best of Both Worlds Western Medicine with Complementary Therapies

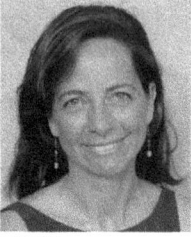

Chapter 2:

Introducing Integrative Medicine – The Best of Both Worlds Western Medicine with Complementary Therapies

Dr Vicki Kotsirilos: Founder of Australasian Integrative Medicine Association (AIMA)

Medicine has developed in leaps and bounds in recent years to include more natural and complementary medicines. What's the connection between mental and physical? I don't want to just put on a band-aide. I want to once and for all get to the root problem for me!

How did the Australasian Integrative Medicine Association (AIMA) come about?

In 1991, Dr Vicki Kotsirilos was working as a GP. I was quite young, I was about 24-25 years of age and I was a new GP who was very much interested in a very holistic approach in my practice, spending extra time with patients and looking at lifestyle factors that we can address to help them out. I was very much interested in natural medicines and the research behind them.

Due to concerns raised by the mainstream profession, I felt it was important to develop an association that would act as a peer body for the medical profession to help build relationships, focus on the evidence and improve communication for this area of health. There was another body called the Australian College of Nutritional and Environmental Medicine that had been training doctors in the area of nutritional and environmental medicine. I called over 200 doctors to organise an urgent meeting and over 100 doctors attended. Consequently, the Australasian Integrative Medicine Association was formed. I became President from the start because I had approached the various organisations and doctors and led this meeting.

In 1991 there was less scientific evidence. In the last 10 years we have seen a large growing body of scientific evidence. We run annual conferences and bring experts in various areas to come and talk about this field and the growing body of science. We are also actively involved with teaching in various universities and at other conferences. We are all pioneers and leaders in our field.

Approximately 70% of consumers use some form of integrated complementary medicine today, and around 30% of General Practitioners regard themselves as integrated medicine practitioners combining the best of orthodox and complementary medicine.

Yes, these are findings from the National Prescriber's Survey completed in October-November 2008. I am a co-author and we did a national survey and also found even the doctors who define themselves as non-integrative, were still using complementary medicine, but to what degree we do not know from the survey.

That's excellent. The AIMA website also has a Practitioner's Directory.

Yes, to find a General Practitioner who integrates complementary medicine.
Go To the AIMA website which is **www.aima.net.au**
Visit the Practitioners Directory and find a doctor that is in your state and area.
It also depends on what your condition is and what is their area of expertise.
The website is also an excellent resource for up-to-date knowledge on complementary medicine.

How would you define stress?

I think stress is how we perceive a situation to be, that may make us feel uncomfortable.

What might be stressful for one person may not be stressful for another person. Stress is how we perceive a situation and generally when we feel uncomfortable.

Stress plays a large role in, and is the basis of, many medical conditions. It appears to be the common cause of relapse towards unhealthy behaviour patterns.

Physiological changes to our body can include increase in heart rate, sweatiness, palpitations, panic attacks, ruminating negative thoughts, being preoccupied by the situation, being concerned by the situation, feeling overwhelmed, feeling that there are no solutions or feeling trapped, feeling uncomfortable, feeling exhausted, tired, etc.

Let's consider hormonal imbalance or biochemical imbalance and pain. What comes first, the biochemical imbalance or the thought?

What comes first is the mind. The mind affects the brain, the brain stimulates the spinal cord, and the spinal nerves hit the adrenals and the endocrine which produce the hormones. That's why the term psycho-neuro-immunology is used. It's usually the psyche, the nervous system, the endocrine system which ultimately affects the immune system. The immune response and the hormone response also give feedback to the brain, this creates a cycle.

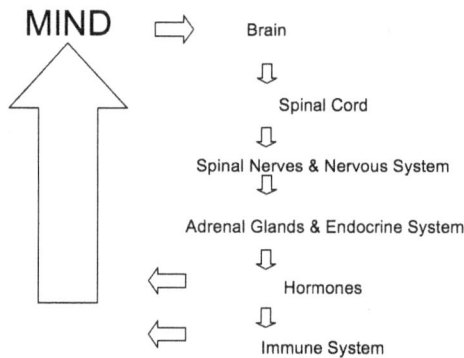

MIND ⟹ Brain

⇩

Spinal Cord

⇩

Spinal Nerves & Nervous System

⇩

Adrenal Glands & Endocrine System

⇩

⟸ Hormones

⇩

⟸ Immune System

This highlights how important it is to start with our mindset.
That's right, as soon as those feelings of discomfort come along, stress etc.- the sooner they are handled, the better, before it goes on to the more chronic physiological states.

Acknowledge there is a problem- Ugghh STRESS!

Where it all starts is acknowledging there is actually a problem.

I actually see a lot of people where you can see this happening. Even the ones I see with disease, sometimes they just don't acknowledge there is a concern.

They are very focused on the end product which is the disease. To acknowledge that one is feeling stressed is a really good place to start even before seeking help. Acknowledging, recognising, that this is ongoing stress and is not right for me.

Good open-ended questions are:

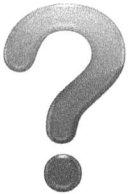

"When did all this start?"

"When did you start to feel unwell?"

"What happened at that time?"

Generally it's not uncommon to find stress precedes an illness "Well actually, I was arguing with my daughter. She wants me to move."

I'm talking about an example of a lady who was in hospital over and over again with diverticulitis. I was seeing her and it was severe and chronic. It was causing her a lot of abdominal pain. I sat her down one day and I asked an open-ended question.

Then it was, "Yes, I was arguing with my daughter and she's not talking to me because she wants me to move up to Queensland and look after her kids and live with her, etc. But I want to stay in Melbourne. I want to stay here and consequently she's not talking to me".

Consequently she had the pain in the belly, the inflammation, the adrenalin, etc.

"Aha I see, that's what's happening."

When we addressed that, that was when we saw real recovery. Her tummy pain subsided. When she came back the following week, she was a lot better. It was also reassuring."Now that explains why you were not getting better. That was behind it."It is the acknowledgement.

This happened quite recently, it's a true story. And it is a very good case example.

There are two aspects here: the Mind and the Body. There is certainly strong scientific evidence today linking the mind and the body. How important is it to have a positive attitude or positive mindset and what is its influence on physical disease?

Yes it's very important. Studies demonstrate that the mind has a direct influence on the physical body. There is good evidence that optimism, hope and a sense of control can improve the quality of a person's life and their health.

When we are feeling more positive and we have a more positive attitude, positive behaviour, positive response, we respond easier to situations that are perceived as stressful or changes in our lives or particular situations.

A positive frame of mind allows us to see things a little bit differently and in a more positive light. We may receive a phone call or have a conversation that might be stressful or upsetting for us, but with a more positive frame of mind we are able to handle it easier.

We are able to think beyond "Now what is the other reason this has happened?" If we are positive about something we might think "Well, maybe it will be fine and everything will be all right. It will sort itself out." We respond to a situation and look for a more positive solution.

If we have a negative frame of mind, where we are challenged or have a conversation that could be unsettling, we will or may perceive it in a negative light and therefore respond much more negatively. Also negative thoughts can make us feel stressed which we know is not good for our health.

I think learning how to be more positive, responding with a much more positive attitude is crucial not just for when we are down and out, but for day-to-day with everything that we come across in life, with everything that we might be challenged by- it might be a conversation- whatever it might be.

The problem with these physiological changes is in the acute setting when our cortisone levels go up, adrenaline levels, heart rate, etc. The body can handle that for short bursts of time.

The problem is when it's ongoing, on a daily basis. It creates wear and tear in our body. It boosts our metabolism. It raises our cortisol.

For example we know cortisol is like giving someone steroids in the long term. It causes problems like osteoporosis, can cause damage of the skin; can cause greying of the hair. It can actually speed up the ageing process of the body.

It is OK for short bursts of time, but not the long-term.

If we keep our adrenalin going, we are eventually going to get exhausted and the body starts to go through a process of wear and tear a lot more rapidly. It accelerates the ageing process, so that's why we don't want to be in that state all the time. It is not good to continue in this state of stress. That's why it's important to address it before we get to that level.

I often think that stress in our lives is a message that something has to change.

Absolutely it is an opportunity for change. We define disease as: "dis" means "un" and "ease" means "comfortable". When the body is diseased, not at ease, it generally means we need to change.

It's the opportunity to change. What we don't want is to be so diseased that it is hard to bring about changes. As soon as there are signs of disease in one's body, that is the first opportunity to think "Hang on, what I'm doing in my life is not right. I need to change."

It's the same with stress causing depression or burnout, fatigue, etc. That would be the end of the line. Before we get to that stage, if we are feeling overly stressed and we recognise that we are not handling the situation, it's so important to recognise we are not at ease. It is the opportunity now to change and bring about for us to feel at ease. To create whatever changes are necessary to feel better.

So what according to you is the first step in tackling daily stress?
Acknowledging it, actually recognising it, being aware is a good start.

And the reason why I say this is because I actually had a patient who presented with chronic muscular pain. She was not acknowledging what was going on behind it at all and that made it really difficult. So the thing is how you do it and how you get them to understand themselves and it might take some time, might take a few consultations. It may not be at the first go, so it's acknowledging beforehand.

It's a simple ABC, A is Accept or Acknowledge, B is Breathe and C is for Change your Mind, Change your Attitude.
Yes, that's excellent.

What evidence can you share on the Power of Love?
Ah, that's very good.

As a clinician and with the work I do day-to-day I think love is crucial.

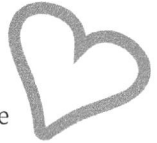

The feeling of love. And this may sound strange, but I love my patients. When I am with my patients I am totally there, I don't think of anything else but them at that moment. I have found, particularly prior to computerising, which only started a year ago, I used to just carry a clipboard and I just looked in their eyes and you feel your heart open, that presence of being there and the feeling of love really helps the healing process.

"And I don't mean "love" like the love we feel with our family members and close loved ones. I mean the "love" we feel like "I love my work", "I love having this patient here", "I love trying to help."
There are many ways we can see "love", so it's important to make this distinction.

The feelings I really more associate with patients would be "caring, empathy, respect", although I do "love my work and having them as my patients"

A lot of old patients say "Lovely to see you. And I say Lovely to see you too!"

In the article "Love Promotes Health" the authors state that love has consequences for health and well-being.

The better we understand the concrete neurobiology of love and its possible secondary implications, the greater is our respect for the significance and potency of love's role in mental and physical health.

Loving-kindness meditation has been used for centuries in the Buddhist tradition to develop love and transform anger into compassion. Positive emotions, compassion and happiness help us to feel better, particularly in stress, and further they improve bodily functions.

Current research on these topics have made the wellness concept evolve from a sometimes esoteric or non-scientific background to become a major focus of progressive medical science.[1]

Love, compassion and joy make our immune system function better and help to battle diseases.

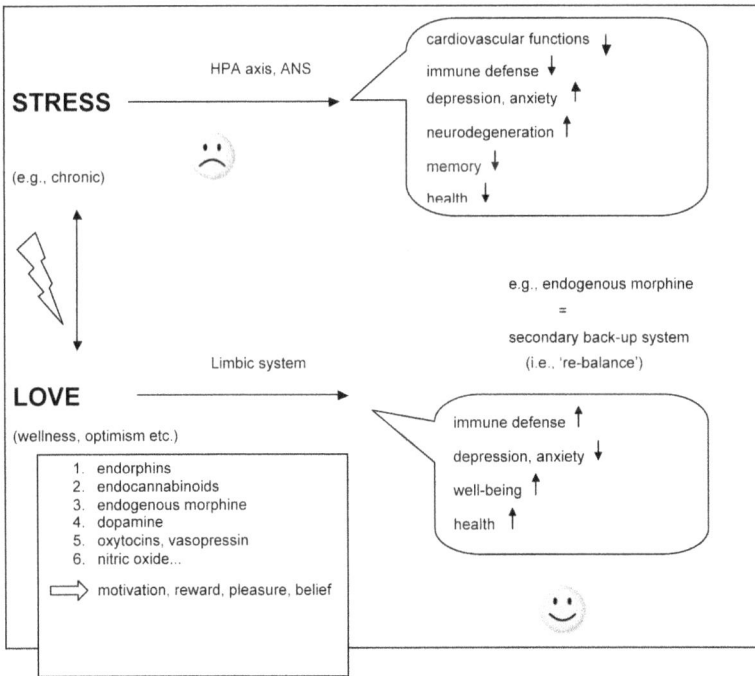

Love and Health. HPA – hypothalamic-pituitary-adrenal (axis); ANS – autonomic nervous system

Source: Love Promotes Health. Tobias Esch & George B. Stefano. Neuroendocrinology Letters No. 3 June Vol.26, 2005 © Neuroendocrinology Letters

Tell me about Joy, Laughter & Meditation

Laughter helps bring on deep relaxation and the release of endorphins bringing on a state of euphoria. Laughter also facilitates deep respiration that increases airflow to the lower parts of the lungs, and like exercise and yoga, laughter can contribute to improvement in health.

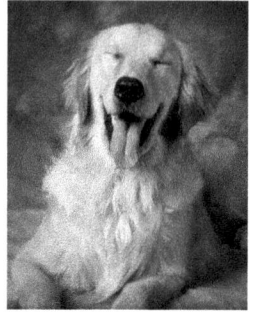

More than 1000 research papers have been published about the positive effects of Meditation.
(Murphy & Donovan, 1997)

It is important to emphasise that patients listen to their bodies and learn to love themselves.

What practical steps would you recommend to patients on a day-to-day basis?

1. Acknowledge the concern.
2. Talk to someone. It might be your trusted, loving, caring GP, or it could be another health practitioner, or it might be people within your own religion. Get it off your chest.
3. Support groups of some kind, spiritual groups, meditation groups.
4. Reading books, self-help books, books on positive thinking. Books like this book.
5. It's good to have role models, people who have experienced stress and have managed it.
6. Find strategies like Cognitive Behavior Therapy.
7. Meditation Retreat, Hindu Retreat, Buddhist Retreat - what ever suits you.
8. Travel, visit local churches – have an open mind to different philosophies, ideas and religions.

Can you tell me 3 things in your life that you are grateful for?

I am so grateful for so many things.
1. One would be the fact that I'm still alive…
2. I am grateful to my spiritual leaders and people who are there to guide me; generally they are wise people with the right advice at the right time…
3. And I'm grateful to have great health and to be loved and to love, like my husband and my children.

Our thoughts, attitudes and beliefs shape our perceptions and our lives, and through various techniques, such as visualising and image techniques, one can change their perceptions and produce profound effects on their physical body and ultimately their health.
(Levine, 1991; Martin & Rossman, 1995; Peterson & Bossio 1995)

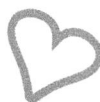

MINDFULNESS MOMENTS FOR TODAY

A - Acknowledge the stress in your life. Areas of discomfort mentally, emotionally, physically.

B – Breathe Deeply and start to be aware of your thoughts. Do nothing with those thoughts. Simply notice what they are. In other words, Be Mindful of your Thoughts.

C – Change something to remove the stress.
Physically change your situation – don't associate with those people again.
Emotionally change the outcome – you choose the positive outcome you want, given the situation you are in.
Mentally change the outcome – your mental attitude will determine how you feel emotionally and physically.

Laugh – borrow a fun video, go to see a fun movie with a friend. I suggest Mary Poppins – it's great fun for all the family!

Smile – Go for a walk down the street and smile to someone you don't know or you do know.

Notice the delight when they smile back, or notice how good you feel even if they don't smile back.

Talk to someone – your neighbour down the street, in a shop, or phone a friend. Notice how much lighter you feel when you don't keep everything bottled up inside of you.

SIMPLE AWARENESS MEDITATION

Sit the body in a chair so that the spine is upright and balanced but relaxed. Have the body symmetrical and allow the eyes to close.

Now, move slowly through each step. Be conscious of the body and its connection with the chair. Feel the feet on the floor. Notice if the feet are tense. If so allow them to relax; let go of the tension. Similarly, be aware of the legs and allow them to relax, and so move up through each part of the body; the stomach, hands, arms, shoulders, neck and face.

Now take in a deep breath and slowly and gently breathe out any tension that remains in the body.
Repeat this twice more, then just allow the breathing to settle into its own natural rhythm without having to control it in any way.

Simply be conscious of the breathing as the air flows in and out of the nose. If thoughts come to your awareness allow them to pass and return the attention to the breathing. There is no need to struggle with the activity of the mind because this simply makes it worse. Don't even wish that it wasn't there; just let go.

After a couple of minutes let the attention move to listening. Hear whatever sounds there are to hear without having to analyse them. Once again, if thoughts come let them pass. If you get distracted by listening to some commentary or chatter in the mind, simply return to the sounds.

At the end of this exercise simply be aware of the body again and then slowly allow the eyes to open.

After settling for a moment quietly move into whatever activities await you.

Stress and Health Implications. Vicki Kotsirilos. Hassad (1996) from Australian Journal of Primary Health – Interchange Vol 4, No.3, 1998

1.Love Promotes Health. Tobias Esch & George B. Stefano. Neuroendocrinology Letters No. 3 June Vol.26, 2005

"Be Master of the Mind rather than Mastered by the Mind"
Zen quote

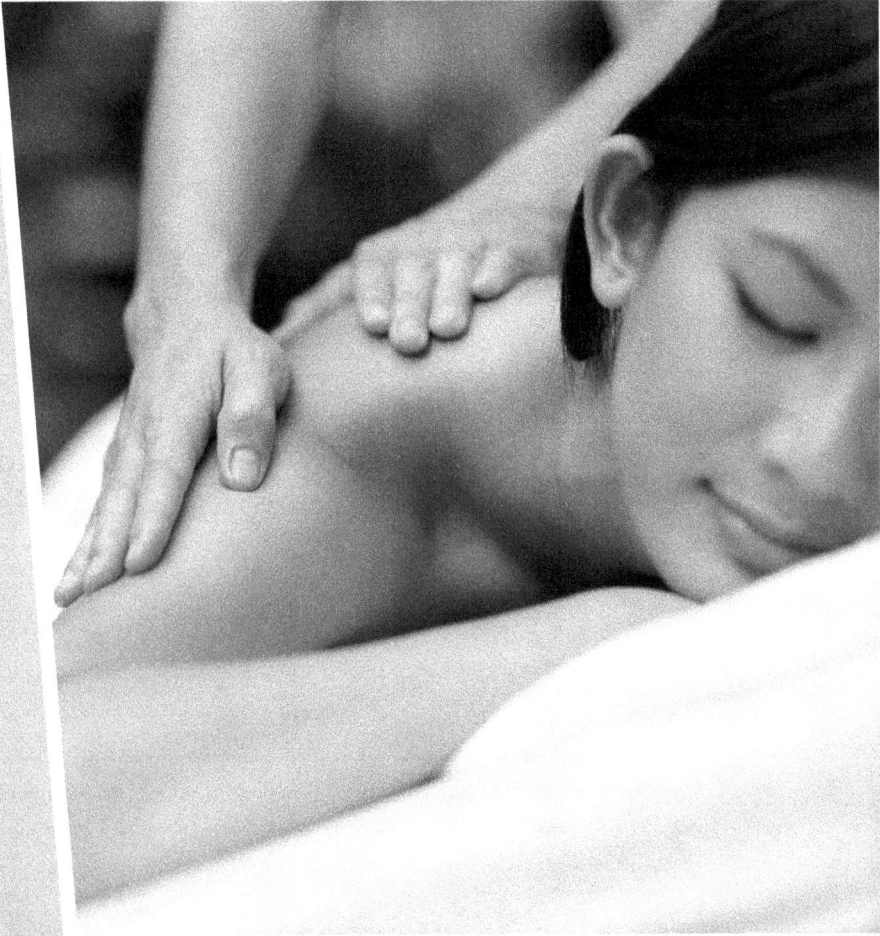

Chapter 3:

The Ayurvedic Approach to Stress & Depression

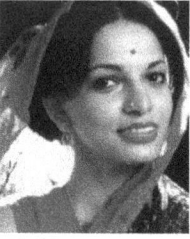

Chapter 3:

The Ayurvedic Approach to Stress & Depression

Shanti Gowans: President Australasian Ayurvedic Practitioners Association. CEO of The Meditation Institute – Southport, Gold Coast, Queensland, Australia

"Sleep is the best meditation."
Dalai Lama

"Your worst enemy cannot harm you as much as your own unguarded thoughts."
Buddhist Quote

Shanti, What is Ayurveda?

Ayurveda is the ancient and extremely well refined traditional medicine of India and one of the oldest healthcare systems in the world. Ayurveda, often regarded as the 'sister' health care system to Yoga, has a recorded history of over 3,000 years.

It is a 'naturopathy' that has come from the wisdom teachings of old, from the Vedas, which are ancient Indian texts.

This naturopathy talks about the holistic nature of life as well as the individual nature of each being. In Ayurveda, the patient or the individual is considered to be the key to healing. According to this ancient science, every person is different and his /her personality is unique.

Thus Ayurveda does not take a 'one size fits all' approach, so what works for one person may not work as well for another and maybe something more unique may work for them. Practice of this knowledge brings health and enlightenment in our daily life.

Health is defined as 'harmony and happiness', hence disease is disharmony and imbalance.

The central principle of Ayurveda is balance, so when this balance is disturbed, we know we are going to experience disease, stress, or both. Daily cycles, seasonal balance- according to Ayurveda, the whole process is linked with the whole package.

The word Ayurveda is comprised of two Sanskrit words 'Ayur' means 'life' and 'Veda' means 'knowledge'. So, it is knowledge about life, a healthy life, a long life. In Ayurveda an average person is expected to live to 120 and if, by chance, there is something like disease in a person's life, then it looks at how to go about making that life better, either by curing that disease or at least managing it.

That's a wonderful life expectation to aim for, 120 years, and to have of beautiful wonderful life on this planet. I think we have the tools here we've just got a bit to learn.

I think, were we living in a more relaxed way, we would probably live a little bit longer. But the process of achievement requires a certain amount of doggedness and so the stress and strain of that sort of living begin to show, which erodes the quality of our lives as well as our health.

People come to Ayurveda for a variety of reasons. Often, people seek out Ayurveda because conventional healthcare has nothing more to offer them, or the treatment options are severe or undesirable. Many people use Ayurveda as a lifetime method of maintaining health and preventing illness. Others use Ayurveda as a complementary healing system in conjunction with other healthcare or health-promoting practices.

Ayurveda is often effective in the treatment of a wide variety of conditions, including: headaches, allergies, chronic fatigue, depression, back pain, digestive disorders, joint pain, menstrual disorders, sleeping problems, asthma, addictions and stress. In the case of life-threatening illnesses such as cancer, AIDS and heart disease, Ayurveda can help improve the quality of life and reduce the side effects of chemotherapy, radiation and medication. In many cases, Ayurveda, in combination with other therapies like yoga and meditation, can halt the progression of a disease.

What is the Ayurvedic approach to disease and in particular, stress?

There are three different manifestations of day-to-day stress from the perspective of Ayurveda - mental, emotional, and physical. Each requires different approaches and therapies.

Mental Stress

Mental stress, according to Ayurveda, is caused by an overuse or misuse of the mind. For instance, if you perform intense mental work many hours a day, or if you work long hours on the computer, it can cause an imbalance in Prana Vata, the mind-body operator concerned with brain activity, energy and the mind.

The first symptom of Prana Vata imbalance is losing the ability to handle day-to-day stress. As the person becomes more stressed, it impacts mental functions such as dhi, dhriti, and smriti - acquisition, retention, and recall. The person's mind becomes hyperactive, yet the person loses the ability to make clear decisions, to think positively, to feel enthusiastic, and even to fall asleep at night.

To address day-to-day mental stress, it is important to begin by managing mental activity. Secondly, you can take measures to pacify Prana Vata, for example, by:
- Favouring Vata-balancing foods, such as sweet, sour, and salty tastes.
- Favouring warm milk and other light dairy products.
- Performing a full-body warm oil self-massage everyday.

It is important to get plenty of rest, and if you are having trouble falling sleep, avoid stimulants like caffeine and sip on herbal tea instead. Relaxing aromatherapy and meditation can help calm the mind.

Chapter 3: *The Ayurvedic Approach to Stress & Depression*

Emotional Stress

Emotional stress can be caused by a problem in a relationship, the loss of a relative, or any situation that might hurt the heart. Emotional stress shows up as irritability, depression, and emotional instability. It affects sleep in a different way than mental stress - it can cause you to wake up in the night and not be able to go back to sleep.

Emotional stress disturbs Sadhaka Pitta, the mind-body operator concerned with the emotions and functioning of the heart. To balance emotional stress, you need to favour Pitta-pacifying foods and routine, such as:

- Eating lots of sweet juicy fruits.
- Favouring Pitta-pacifying foods such as the sweet, bitter and astringent tastes.
- Drinking a cup of warm milk with cooling rose petal preserve before bed.
- Cooking with cooling spices such as cardamom, coriander, cilantro, and mint.
- A daily self-massage with a cooling oil such as coconut oil.
- **Going to bed before 10:00 p.m.**

Physical Stress

Physical stress is caused by misuse or overuse of the body, such as exercising too much or working for extended periods at a job that is physically taxing. This can cause a person to experience physical fatigue, along with mental fogginess, difficulty in concentrating, and dullness of the mind.

Excessive physical strain causes three sub-doshas to go out of balance: Shleshaka Kapha, the subdosha concerned with lubrication of the joints and moisture balance in the skin, Vyana Vata, which governs the circulation, nerve impulses and the sense of touch, and Tarpaka Kapha, which governs the neuro humors.

Another reason for physical stress can be too little exercise, which results in a sluggish digestion and the formation of ama, the digestive impurities that clog the channels. In either type of physical fatigue, the process of regenerating cells slows down, and thus the cells themselves become physically tired.

The solution is to balance Vata and to support Kapha to make the body more stable and nurturing, for example, by:
• Getting adequate rest and moderate exercise.
• Following a Vata-Kapha pacifying diet.
• Performing the full-body warm oil self massage everyday.

Certain foods are natural stress busters according to Ayurveda. These include walnuts, almonds, coconut, sweet, juicy, seasonal fruit such as pears, apples (cooked if possible), milk, and fresh cheeses such as panir or ricotta.

On the other hand, if you build your resilience to stress through natural methods, you can begin to experience stressors more as a challenge or a positive opportunity for growth. If you learn to evoke the 'stay and play' rather than the 'fight or flight' response, you can truly live a stress-free life of self-actualization, and become a 'spiritual being' in human form.

Note: Vata, Pitta and Kapha are the three psycho-physiological Ayurvedic principles that govern all the activities of the mind and body. A person enjoys perfect health if these principles are in perfect balance.

Introducing Ayurvedic Philosophy

According to Ayurveda's understanding of the creation of the cosmos, in the beginning (which means before anything else), emptiness dances; this dance is wind and wind is seen to be erratic and to cause friction. Then heat, and the action of the heat upon the nothingness, sweats the universe into existence and as the liquid portion cools, it encrusts itself and coheses and we have the cosmic dance now in five steps.

Stillness, movement, transformation, fluidity and cohesion then morph themselves into the five universal elements which are known as space, air, fire, water and earth. We now have two sets here, the wave and the particle. According to Ayurveda everything in the manifested universe has its origin in these. Healing replicates creation.

Chapter 3: *The Ayurvedic Approach to Stress & Depression*

The tool that is probably the most relevant for all of us, and is the easiest to access, is the breath, because here we are talking about the wind element. The breath is the link between the intangible world (of the spirit) and the tangible world (of the cell).

Now, the combination of these five elements creates something which is known as Ayurveda dosha. Dosha means 'fault'. The combination of space and air, where space represents stillness and air represents movement. The two are kind of incompatible but through some fault they come together, creating vata dosha which is like the biological principle of wind.

The combination of fire and water, which again are incompatible, through some fault come together creating pitta dosha- the principle of transformation. The combination of water and earth create an amalgam called kapha dosha. On the micro cell level everything is made out of three elements known as vata (air), pitta (fire) and kapha (earth). Our body is also made out of millions of cells and each cell contains these three elements. The level of each element varies from person to person and that is what makes the differences in our personalities. So various combinations of these three doshas are like the signature tune for each person. All of us have some quantity and quality of all of these three which is like our thumbprint, our constitutional blueprint and for us to be balanced we need to be as close to our constitutional blueprint as we experienced at conception.

When we veer away from our constitutional thumbprint we experience stress and disease. So, for instance, according to the principles in Ayurveda, like increases like: if a Vata person is exposed to excessive movement or wind it will increase their Vata, whereas if they are exposed to the opposite principle it will bring their Vatta down. If a Pitta person is exposed to more heat it will increase the Pitta quality in them, so what was originally their constitution, might now even become an imbalance for them until they come back to the thumbprint, their signature constitution from birth.

Imbalance causes physical symptoms?

Yes, together with a mental and emotional breakdown. Even though we all are born with more influence of one or a combination of these elements, from time to time it changes according to the age, seasons, life situations, food intake, thoughts, etc. The perfect health is a state of mind and body in equilibrium. Disease is the result of imbalance in these three doshas (elements) in the body.

From the Ayurvedic perspective when you balance these three different constitutions, you are then closer to this blueprint. This impacts the physical, mental and emotional and heals in a natural way because we are working with the natural elements, as well as those elements in nutrition and the foods we eat.

Yes, because when we look at what those elements represent, we don't just talk about the air that we breathe, air represents something beyond that. It is that quality of movement which has no substance which is present in the food we eat and in everything else; the quality of movement is present in every cell, so it is present in the movement of the blood flowing through the body, in the movement of our thoughts.

The fire quality doesn't just represent fire in the universe like the sun or fire in the body, but is a part of the transformation and heat in the body and represents even our ability to digest information. In the universe, the microcosm and the macrocosm represent each other and the universe outside is also reflected within each human body.

What is the first step you recommend when someone comes to you with stress in their life?

Stress and pain are shadows of the outstretched hand of the divine. It is the universal Truth asking us to make a change that will help us fulfil the purpose of our life.

When people approach us with stress, we first would ascertain what dosha they are, what their signature tune is, because to bring them back to that would be to bring them back to the optimum tune that they play.

Chapter 3: *The Ayurvedic Approach to Stress &*
Depression

**Go to www.HowToOvercomeStressNaturally.com/Resources
to fill in the Ayurvedic Dosha Questionnaire, to find your
signature tune.**

For instance, a vata dosha person under stress would get anxious and
nervous and fearful.

A pitta person under stress would get angry and aggressive.

A kapha person under stress would go into a kind of state of no action
like a paralysis that is the precursor to depression.

When we find out what their constitution is- which we find out when
we go through a series of observations and questioning- and they talk
about how they feel things they then begin to understand their own
characteristic state.

> **It's really an explanation and education as to why we
> wouldn't want them to be anything but who they are, to
> honour who they are. To function optimally, they must be
> who they are.**

With vata constitutions, we would understand why they are anxious
and fearful and firstly we look at food being the first medicine we give
them. So we want food that will nourish vata, to help overcome the
sense of fear and instability in vata and ground them with a bit more
earth principle.

Pitta people are already fiery and are getting to the point where they
are short fused. As anger is predominant we want to reduce the heat,
so we would balance them out with cooling foods.

Kapha people are too cool and too slow, so we want to change that and
increase a little bit of fire in their systems and bring some space and air
into them. We would do this trough the medium of food, introducing
these elements through their nourishment and nutrition.

Ayurveda does recommend stimulation of all the senses too, for
instance touch and massage- not necessarily having it done by an
external source, but self massage with the use of appropriate products

that will help balance the particular Dosha. For vata dosha we would want something that's a little bit more grounding, heavier, like heating oil. For kapha dosha that's already heavy, we would want something lighter or perhaps no oil at all.

The first step is in gaining a better understanding of ourselves, understanding where we are at, how we are reacting, and then simply to redress the imbalance using these Ayurvedic principles.

There are so many people I have met who feel so bad about who they are and how they feel, and this is unnecessary. What if we could entertain the possibility that there was nothing wrong with this person? Yoga understands the difference between fixing and healing. Yoga recognises that the human condition can never be fixed; only healed. When we try to fix our lives through getting rid of grief, loss, or anguish – anything we don't want- we are simply re-arranging our confusion. We hope to find a better place, a better state of mind, than the one we are currently experiencing. We never get to the root of our fundamental dissatisfaction. Healing challenges our ability to accommodate experience rather than trying to live around it. It challenges us to participate in the unravelling of our own personal mystery.

Ayurveda and Yoga are so welcoming to everything and that's what acceptance is all about. There is absolutely no reason to reject anything. In a holistic perspective, life is an all-inclusive oneness and it allows us to negotiate with it.

For anybody who wishes to adopt Ayurveda in their life and help others with this natural science, unveiling the secrets of ancient Ayurveda teaches traditional methods of self diagnosing. The skin is the largest organ in the body and it reflects most of our health problems, even from very initial stages. Our eyes, tongue, teeth, nails etc. are the primary diagnosing mediums for the body.

We can also learn to examine our sweat, urine, stools and daily mental functions that are the base cause of most of our health/disease symptoms.

Chapter 3: *The Ayurvedic Approach to Stress & Depression*

The three guidelines of traditional Ayurveda are food, life style and thoughts (aahar, vihar and vijar). To maintain a healthy body and mind it is very important to take care of yourself with the right food, a disciplined lifestyle and a balanced mind with healthy thoughts.

A disciplined lifestyle means giving our body the proper rest and exercise. According to traditional Ayurveda, proper sleep is the base of health and sleep is known as the best therapy in life.

Sleep, like most healthy and beautiful things on this earth, is free. The only thing we need to do is to fix an appointment with our bed and keep it every day.

Traditional Ayurveda explains the need for everybody to have a personal lifestyle and food structure. We all are born with a different body/mind structure and our physical organs and mental functions are related to it.

That means we all are unique and need more specific design in making our own lifestyle.

In addition to sleep, the other most important part in our life is exercise. A proper exercise maintains our health by keeping the body in the right balance, with strength and flexibility throughout all our years. It also keeps positive energies in our body and mind and keeps us away from pains and aches throughout all seasons.

Yoga is a perfect daily exercise for our body and mind, as long as we know the right asanas (postures) according to our dosha (body/mind type). Elementary yoga works upon the five universal elements that are present in our body in the basic doshas: air, fire and water known as vata, pitta and kapha. We are different in our body because of the five elements and three doshas, and this difference impacts the earth, sun and moon effect upon us.

The eight limbs of classical yoga of course, offer more than just different contortionist postures and include a blueprint for spiritual growth. They include appropriate guidelines for discipline, conduct, exercise, breathing, control of the senses, concentration, meditation and self realisation.

People approach yoga at all different levels. Sometimes when people come to yoga they come in - and keep in mind, how we do one thing is how we do everything - with the street savvy garden variety speed, at which we approach life.

Then as we are willing to get deeper into yoga, we take it past the mere physical exercise component, into something that is deeper for us, into metaphysical levels.

Then yoga becomes not just exercise, it is then more like having a shower. What showering does to the outer body, is what yoga does internally too, it cleanses the body inside and out. Body and mind are inseparably contained within each other. The friction of one makes the movements of the other. This is how yoga helps to calm the mind; by keeping the body still in an asana (position) and vice versa.

Outer yoga is concerned about strengthening the musculo-skeletal system; your joints, muscles, tendons, bones and spinal column. Shanti yoga works all the muscle groups through a series of stretches and poses that are held for periods of time, whilst breathing.

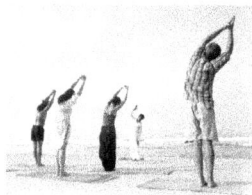

The best thing about yoga, as opposed to the gym or weight training, is that you have to use your own body.

This makes you really aware of all the connections in your body and how to balance yourself. It helps you develop patience and manage stress.

Having more access to our bodies is a pre-requisite for us to learn how to meditate properly. You will become physically and mentally stronger. The healing wisdom of Shanti yoga helps you emerge fortified with inner-peace and a deeper understanding of life.

Inner yoga deals with nourishing the internal organs and cultivating prana, or internal energy. Practice promotes intuitive intelligence, energy, serenity and focus. For this to be possible, techniques of digesting toxins, tendon changing, marrow washing and self-massage of internal organs must be the focus and be practiced.

These classes incorporate the Upper back, Neck and Shoulder series; Lower back, Sacrum and Hips series; Core strength and Lower body series; Serpent in the Spine series and Body of Light series. In addition, students practice the postures of standing yoga.

Yoga explores the five elements (earth, water, fire, wind and space), which are the basic constituents of both our bodies and the environment.

The vegetable and animal (including reptile and aquatic) forms of yoga represent the earth dance together with the water dance which strengthens tendons and bones, preserving generative energy.

The bird forms of yoga represent sky dance and help improve our sense of balance and enhance our agility.

The rishi forms represent the road to enlightenment.

The deva forms represent instructions in the immortals' guide to self-healing and breath regulation;

and the **cosmic forms** represent the primordial limitlessness.

In remedial yoga, most people need to heal. That does not mean we're necessarily sick; to heal simply means to be whole. In remedial and healing yoga there is no judgment, there are no standards, just encouragement.

If people understand that this is part of the process which is so natural, then they are far ahead in the whole process.

Then we can laugh and have fun, not the hehe haha type of laughing, but genuinely connect to that bliss that is part of being alive.

Approach life no matter what happens in a balanced way. That's the key to maintain balance, especially in the world today, when there is so much upheaval and change. How do we maintain that balance within?

The Buddha called change impermanence. When we struggle with this notion of impermanence, it's because of our habits of attachment and revulsion. It is our mindset and resistance to go with acceptance, to go with the flow, the flow of the universe.

If we are fighting the universe, then we are going to experience some stress. This is not necessarily a bad thing because according to Vedic (yoga and Ayurveda) philosophy there is no good or bad, as everything comes from the one. So what appears good or bad is simply relative to the situation and is just part of a learning curve that will hopefully enable us to come to our own resolutions about how to come back to that sense of being balanced.

How can we ride the waves of change in life around us without feeling stressed?

Meditation is where it's at. The simple yet profound practice of mindfulness-awareness meditation enables us to look precisely at our state of mind without altering it. This practice cultivates openness toward ourselves and our environment, moment by moment.

When we practice openness, our lives can be a journey of wakeful and genuine existence. The effort and training in meditation allows us to relax into unconditional trust, bringing a sense of freedom and space.

> **This is the purpose of meditation, to awaken in us the sky-like nature of mind and to introduce us to that which we really are, our unchanging pure awareness, which underlies the whole of life and death.**

In the stillness and silence of meditation, we glimpse and return to that deep inner nature that we have so long ago lost sight of amid the busy-ness and distraction of our minds.

Chapter 3: *The Ayurvedic Approach to Stress & Depression*

Shanti, what inspires you at the start of each day?

My day starts with meditation, yoga and pranayama.

How can people find an Ayurvedic practitioner in their local area?

You can get in touch with one of the associations. There are several. Ours is the Ayurvedic Practitioner's Association. http://www.ayurvedapractitionersaustralia.com/

Ayurveda is a very new field in Australia and in the Western world in general, although it's such an ancient science from the East. I wouldn't even like to say that it's Indian, though a few Indians might get annoyed with me for saying this, but I think it belongs to the world.

While India might be where Ayurveda originated, as it is a gift to the whole world, to say that Ayurveda belongs only to Indians is like saying that Einstein's theory of relativity belongs only to the Jews.

Could you tell us about The Meditation Institute on the Gold Coast in Queensland?

The Meditation Institute is a spiritual centre for the study and practice of yoga, meditation and Ayurveda. I founded it in 1972 and still give regular teachings in Yoga, Vedanta, Buddhism, Ayurveda and classes in yoga and meditation. The Meditation Institute is a highly-respected, private Registered Training Organisation (R.T.O. 30834) compliant with National and State Government Quality Standards for education and training.

At The Meditation Institute we run two centres, a city centre in Southport called Shanti Yoga and our eco-meditation, wellness retreat centre in Beachmont. The retreat is on 70 acres of dairy farm and rain forest and we can house 18 people at the moment. It's absolutely stunning. At the retreat centre we have spring water, milk from the farm across the road and solar heating. The rooms are individual, so it's like having your own capsule. Our retreat centre is called Nirvana. It's a Wellness Meditation Retreat and is designed along ecological lines.

You can learn more about the Nirvana Wellness Retreat by logging onto **www.shantiyoga.com.au.**

At our Southport centre, we have daily classes in yoga, meditation, deep relaxation and yoga breathing that support everyday commuters and urban people's lifestyles. We also offer children's classes. We run a course called yogability, which is for disabled people aged between 18-30 years and also cater for mature aged people in our classes. The approach is gentle and healing. Yoga is not about being a contortionist.

In yoga, the breath is the key. It drives everything and now it is recognised that there is a system of meridians in the body, which are definite pathways of energy, which in yoga is known as prana, some may be familiar with the Chinese term for it which is chi.

In yoga we talk about balance, so we go back to balance and its energy which is a combination of Yin and Yang. In Yoga we know this as the solar and the lunar flows of energy. Sometimes we might excess and end up with too much solar or too much lunar energy, or you could say too much yin or yang.

The idea in Yoga is to be whole, to be balanced with both flows with the breath being the key, that kind of washes out the marrow and the tendons at the internal level, allowing the outer body to redress itself. We work with form, of course, in Yoga, but there are also the aspects of fuel and flow.

Meditation is the spiritual essence of yoga. Through meditation we can start to bring into our lives greater understanding of who we are, our purpose for being here and where real happiness lies. Meditation provides insights into the workings of the mind and emotions. It further helps you develop clarity and wisdom, gaining a greater understanding of life. The art of meditation has been practiced by saints and sages to bring about the joyful state of self-realisation. In this consciousness a person is free from temporary worries, anxieties and concerns and is immersed in a higher spiritual happiness and inner peacefulness.

Chapter 3: *The Ayurvedic Approach to Stress & Depression*

If someone is not in a yoga class but in a stressful situation in daily life, can simply taking a deep breath make a difference?

Yes, huge. Even if your whole world is falling to pieces, just stop and breathe. Breathe in, then breathe out. Breathe. When you just come back to centre you are so much more able to address what's happening. The whole idea is not to run away and hide. Sometimes we might do this when we are under stress but the whole idea is to be kind and brave in the world.

All our lives represent the hero's journey and it's how we overcome whatever we need to do in a heroic way. It doesn't mean being foolhardy or anything, it means being noble including being noble about ourselves. As you know, I have written a book about breath. It's called Breathe for Health and I've also produced a CD with breathing practices in it called Breathe for Health.

Breathing techniques allow the body to relax and let go of tension, enhancing one's ability to deal with stressful situations. These techniques deeply rejuvenate the whole body; you will feel fresh and enlivened. Because of the connection between the breath, the emotions and the mind ("just take a deep breath and relax") your mind calms and becomes clearer and more focused. I now run a special breath class called pranayama, which is a class dedicated to an hour of breathing practices.

That's a great incentive to go and visit the Gold Coast. Do you come down to Melbourne?

Yes, I come down to Melbourne a few times a year and run a weekend workshop of Yoga. It's yoga from the ground up, namely Yoga, meditation, breathwork and nourishment with the philosophical kind of grounding that all of this comes from.

Is there anything else you would like to share with us to help lead a stress free life?

The biggest thing is meditation. I know people struggle with it, partly because some people confuse it with religion and sometimes it is confronting with all this frenetic stuff going on in our heads.

However, you will never regret taking up the practice of meditation. It's a step-by-step process that allows you to bring your mind home, not the mind of belief but the mind of clarity.

It is about sitting down and being present, connecting with that sense of presence that isn't separated from us. You know, the universe comes into being when you are born.

And can you have a meditative movement any time during the day?

The ideal understanding of meditation is mindfulness, being present, and it is hard for us to be present when we are stressed as we tend to fight or flight. The fight is just the mirror fighting the image but really the witnesser stands outside both and that's what we cultivate in meditation, the witnesser. The running and hiding stuff is all about our escape routes that we use, which is why we are so distracted and this doesn't help us in our lives, our work or in anything.

In meditation we talk about the universe and come to understand that there is a tender stillness that exists in the mind. Thoughts are like clouds in the sky, they obscure the clarity of the sky. When we come to that clear sky of mind, we see that we are the universe. It is really something we come to embrace as our fundamental reality and it is seamless.

This obscuration is what holds us with a separated sense of being; me against the world.

Ultimately it is separation at the root of so many problems.
This is the ignorance that Buddha talked about.

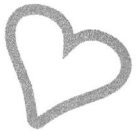

As opposed to love which is cohesive, all embracing and one.
Love is so freeing and it's this separation which brings about attachment which is the opposite of love; it's like a prison.

Chapter 3: *The Ayurvedic Approach to Stress & Depression*

Shanti, what are 3 things you are grateful for in your life?

1. I am grateful for the path that I have never swerved off and all that it's enabled me to offer countless other people.
2. I'm grateful to my husband, who is the nicest person I have ever come across and after 36 years of marriage he has offered me such kind, wonderful friendship and support.
3. I am grateful for my dog. I think she is in the same category as my husband. We have the kind of relationship issues that allow us to function well in the world.

It's quite difficult, because I'm grateful for everything. I'm grateful for every moment that I breathe.

Then, when I look around I wonder what is there not to be celebrated, in spite of all the chaos and terrible things that are happening. There are so many people in need of healing.

The world needs more smiles, not sighs. Breathing in, say 'yes'. Breathing out say 'thank you'.

POWER ACTIONS FOR TODAY

1. FIRST UPON WAKING - PRANAYAMA
Long Deep Breathing.
As you lie in bed, eyes closed, start your day with deep, long, relaxed breathing.
Take a long deep breath, blowing your belly outwards as you inhale.
Exhale and Let Go. Surrender.
Deep Breath In and say"Yes", Exhale slowly and say"Thank you".
Deep Breath In and say"Yes", Exhale slowly and say"Thank you".
Repeat for 5-10 minutes to energise your body and clear your mind to begin your day.

2. Remember foods that are natural STRESS busters are walnuts, almonds, coconut, sweet juicy, seasonal fruit such as pears, apples (cooked if possible), milk, and fresh cheeses such as panir or ricotta. Have a snack throughout the day.

3. Give Yourself a Nurturing Massage: neck and shoulders, your feet, or wherever your body is calling out for attention. Do this for at least 5 minutes. Even better if you have a friend you can swap with.

SIMPLE DAILY MINDFULNESS / AWARENESS

At the START of your day take a few moments to
STILL THE MIND.
Be Mindful. Be Aware. Observe the monkey chatter of the mind. Watch
thoughts come and go.

Sit comfortably, spine straight, feet and legs uncrossed.
Close your eyes, take a DEEP BREATH IN. As you exhale LET GO.
LET GO of all thoughts; LET them drift away.
Take another DEEP BREATH IN, simply be aware that thoughts are
passing through your mind. You are not attaching to those thoughts. You
have no need for those thoughts right now, you simply observe them.
As you exhale LET GO even further, LET GO and RELAX, LET GO of
everything.
Take another DEEP BREATH IN, and notice the stillness that exists as
thoughts drift away.
You are left experiencing a stillness and peacefulness of Mind.
Exhale and be aware of the Openness and Freedom you have.
Your Mind is calm and aware. There is only the breath. Nothing else is
important.
Now slowly open your eyes and maintain this stillness.
Take a few long deep breaths, remaining calm and still.
Still allowing any thoughts to drift away. You pay no attention to
thoughts.
Notice the calm, still, peace, warmth and love of your being.
Focus your attention on your heart. Breathe deeply.
Know you can always return to this place of calm, still, peace, warmth
and love- simply breathe deeply and focus on your heart. It is as
simple as that. In time, that sense will grow and serve you well in
health and happiness.

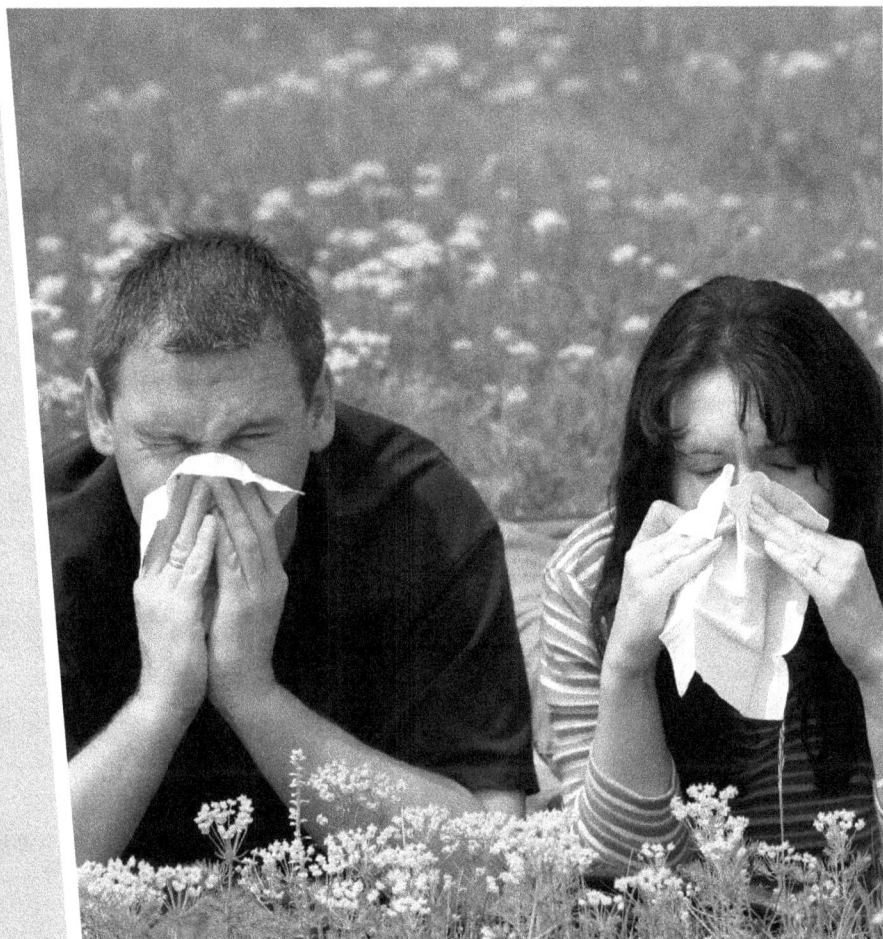

Chapter 4:

Nutrition Healing - Vitamins, Minerals, Fatty Acids and Mental Health

Chapter 4:

Nutrition Healing - Vitamins, Minerals, Fatty Acids and Mental Health

Blake Graham, B.Sc (Honours): Clinical Nutritionist, Director of Nutritional Healing Western Australia

Blake, please tell us about your background and Nutritional Healing.

I became passionate about the role diet can play in our health 10 years ago. My interests have since expanded to a wider range of health areas, e.g. the role of toxic chemicals, mind-body medicine, etc. I acquired a B.Sc (Honours) in nutrition from Curtin University, ACT, and did my honours thesis researching nutritional and metabolic aspects of chronic fatigue syndrome (CFS).

www.nutritional-healing.com.au

I run a health clinic in Perth, Western Australia specialising in science based, non-drug treatments for chronic medical issues.

One of my key interests is mental health and I see many people with depression, anxiety, bipolar disorder and schizophrenia. Plus many highly stressed people. It's become clear to me that stress is a huge problem in itself, plus it can exacerbate just about any health issue.

What is Nutritional and Environmental Medicine?

Nutritional Medicine is the therapeutic use of nutrients and diet to treat health problems. This could take the form of a variety of avenues. For example, a person with depression could be found to be deficient in magnesium which is exacerbating their symptoms. A second use is using a nutrient in a therapeutic manner, rather than simply correcting an obvious deficit.

For example, high doses of omega-3 fatty acids (e.g. fish/flax oil) can have a potent influence on lowering inflammation and treating medical conditions related to inflammation.

People may find they have a food intolerance (e.g. dairy/eggs) which is contributing to their heath problem.

A basic way to view the importance of diet in regards to our chronic health problems is in terms of the levels of essential nutrients (vitamins, minerals, protein, healthy fats) our diet provides. While this issue is certainly important, the influence of diet goes well beyond this.

Various aspects of diet influence virtually every contributing factor in chronic illness. Diet can be seen as one therapeutic tool to modulate the mechanisms behind disease.

Mechanisms of illness modulated by diet:
  i.   Inflammation
  ii.   Oxidative Stress
  iii. Intestinal micro-organism balance
  iv.   Detoxification
  v.   Hormone/neurochemical balance
  vi.   Intake of toxic chemicals
  vii. Immune function
  viii. Circadian rhythm
  ix.   Food intolerances
  x.   Genetic expression

Environmental Medicine is a branch of alternative medicine/complementary medicine which identifies and treats the environmental factors contributing to our health issues. This includes environmental exposures such as toxic metals (e.g. mercury), pesticides, electromagnetic field (EMF), inhalant allergies (e.g. dust) and toxic mould.

There is a strong overlap between nutritional and environmental medicine and they generally co-exist. They both relate to the idea of treating issues causing symptoms, rather than merely suppressing symptoms. My favourite term is actually integrative medicine. Integrative medicine combines the best that both conventional and alternative/complementary medicine has to offer.

No one modality (e.g. herbal medicine or pharmaceutical medicine) has all the answers. The best approach is to choose from a wide array of options as appropriate given the individual circumstances.

Conventional medicine is brilliant in dealing with acute emergency situations. For example, if I had bacterial meningitis I would want IV antibiotics, not Echinacea and vitamin C.

But for dealing with issues like chronic stress and chronic fatigue states, less conventional options are generally the better avenue.

Can you tell us about the relationship between nutrition, the environment and stress?

There are many influences on our stress levels. Nutrition and environment are two of many.

When a person has high stress levels the best approach is not simply to try one modality (e.g. nutrition) and then another (e.g. Tai Chi), but to openly consider which approaches may be best for their personal situation.

Ideally all the basic requirements for good health should be addressed simultaneously; nutrition, sleep, rest, exercise, clean environment, etc.

Best results come from a full picture look at health rather than dabbling here and there, trying to find a solution.

Get the basics done first and then look at more advanced therapeutic options.

For example, if you only get two hours sleep and live off coffee, then just taking vitamins or meditating is not going to cut it. These basic considerations are non-negotiable.

Chapter 4: *Nutrition Healing - Vitamins, Minerals, Fatty Acids and Mental Health*

Nutrition can relate to stress in a wide variety of ways.

Dietary choices can both lower levels of our natural relaxing/calming neurochemicals (e.g. serotonin/endorphins/GABA) and increase levels of anxiety increasing neurochemicals (e.g. adrenalin).

The chemical in our brain raised by most anti-depressants, serotonin, and the chemical target of many anxiety medications, GABA, are both made from nutrients. They are made from amino acids.

Serotonin is made from tryptophan and GABA is made from glutamine.

In fact when scientists want to study the effects of serotonin deficiency they feed people a few tryptophan devoid meals. Under these conditions they find decreased mood, increased urge to drink alcohol, decreases in elation, vigour and friendliness. This is just one of many similar examples. These chemicals in our brain also require various vitamins and minerals for their production.

Our brain chemistry balance relates strongly to our nutrient status.

Deficiencies of certain nutrients are much more common than you might think.

Our modern diet and food processing methods are extremely different to those during the period in which we evolved.

A variety of other factors lower nutrient levels: stress, medications, absorption problems, genetics, toxic chemicals, etc.

The notion we can get all the nutrients we need from diet actually applies to some people but not others.

The symptoms of most nutrient deficiencies actually include a lot of brain related symptoms. Symptoms such as nervousness, mild depression, behavioural changes, irritability, insomnia and others are all very common when looking over the symptoms of low nutrient levels.

For example, low vitamin D levels- extremely common- have been linked with seasonal affective disorder (SAD) and other forms of depression. This partly relates to their role in producing neurochemicals and partly to other issues.

Eating refined sugar produces a surge of insulin and stress hormones (cortisol and adrenalin). This puts a great stress on our hormonal system and promotes inflammation.

Caffeine is documented to increase anxiety levels. One study found aspartame (e.g. in diet soft drinks) exacerbated symptoms in those with depression.

There are countless other examples, too many to list here. In a nutshell poor dietary choices and nutrient imbalances alter our physical/chemical balance making us less resilient to stress and lowering our stress threshold.

Environmental exposures often cause symptoms relating to mood and brain function. For example, mercury causes symptoms of depression, insomnia, irritability, restlessness, memory impairment, poor concentration and fatigue.

As these symptoms are very non-specific they are often attributed to other things, such as stress or a person's general nature.

What is the greatest nutritional imbalance you see in people who are stressed?

Among people with high stress levels magnesium deficiency is extremely common.

High stress levels actually lower levels of magnesium and low magnesium levels cause symptoms such as irritability, anxiousness, agitation, poor mood and insomnia. So it is a vicious cycle. If the imbalance came before or after your current life stressor, either way you are better without it. The following is a list of magnesium deficiency symptoms:

- Muscle cramps, spasms or pain (e.g. back ache, neck ache, leg/foot cramps)
- Muscle tension
- Muscle twitches, tics or jerks
- Muscle weakness
- Mild muscle tremor
- Restless legs
- Fatigue / sighing
- Breathlessness / chest tightness
- Heart palpitations / arrhythmias
- Numbness or tingling of skin or "creepy-crawly" feeling under skin
- Sensitivity to loud noises or sudden bright light
- Headaches / migraines
- Menstrual cramps / pain
- Teeth grinding (bruxism)
- Frequent constipation or anal spasms
- Difficulty falling asleep or frequent nocturnal awakenings
- Irritable, anxious, agitated, depressed or panic attacks

All vitamins and minerals are involved in one or more biochemical pathways and/or physiological actions which influence the function of the human brain.

Most vitamin and mineral deficiencies result in psychiatric symptoms in a significant number of people, and in people with psychiatric diagnoses these deficiencies are often associated with more severe symptoms and result in poorer outcomes from conventional treatment.

What sort of tests do you conduct to determine imbalances in the body?

It depends on the situation and the person's interest in doing tests.

I use a detailed questionnaire (16 pages/7000+ words) I have developed and refined since 2002.

I start by looking over this and talking to the person, trying to gauge which issues are likely to be relevant to them and which issues are most likely of high importance given their health goals. On one end of the spectrum I do zero testing for some people, while for people with very serious health issues I do extensive laboratory testing, choosing from the following options:

i.	Stool microbiology (bacteria/yeast/parasites)
ii.	Urine heavy metals
iii.	Hair mineral analysis
iv.	Blood fatty acids
v.	Salivary adrenal hormone profile
vi.	Functional liver detoxification profile
vii.	Urine organic acid testing (OAT)
viii.	Blood amino acid testing
ix.	Serum copper and ceruloplasmin
x.	Urine iodine
xi.	IgG food intolerance testing
xii.	Urine kryptopyrroles ('pyroluria')
xiii.	MELISA metal hypersensitivity
xiv.	MTHFR (folate metabolism) gene test

These tests investigate metabolic, nutritional, toxic, genetic, gastrointestinal and hormonal influences on our mental health.

What are the latest developments on how environmental factors affect health?

Research on the influence of electromagnetic radiation (EMR) on our health is both fascinating and concerning.

Chapter 4: *Nutrition Healing - Vitamins, Minerals, Fatty Acids and Mental Health*

While people with vested interests in believing otherwise play down the impact EMR can have on our health, evidence is accumulating that there is reason for great concern.

Long term (e.g. 20 years+) influence of daily mobile phone use has of course not been studied for obvious reasons.

Some experts suspect this could contribute to neurodegenerative diseases.

Headsets using air-filled wireless tubes can easily overcome this problem. Mobile phones are only one of many sources of EMR.

For example some people have high exposures from sleeping in close proximity to their meter box.

EMR is known to lower melatonin levels and impair sleep. It is also documented that certain individuals are overly sensitive to the influence of EMR which can cause symptoms such as tingling, fatigue, sleep problems, headaches, dizziness and concentration problems.

www.emfacts.com is an excellent website people can visit for more information.

I have recently been doing a lot of reading about sensitivities to metals and the impact this can have on our health. A lot of people are immunologically reactive or sensitive to certain metals, the most common being nickel.

Nickel is found in some earrings, foods and other sources. This can contribute to many health issues, including chronic fatigue.

Other people might be sensitive to gold, mercury, palladium and titanium. I have recently started using a test called the MELISA test (www.melisa.org/) which assesses for metal sensitivities.

Evidence has now piled up that heavy metals such as mercury, lead and aluminium contribute to neurological disorders such as Alzheimer's and autism.

In your opinion, what is the fundamental cause of (negative) stress? There are external triggers for stress but why does one person respond one way and someone else another way?

Stress is highly multi-factored. To the person experiencing stress the cause seems obvious, the external situation. However stress is more about our reaction to external events. Some people feel stressed for no reason.

What determines our reaction to events? A combination of our physical/biological balance and psycho-social factors such as the cognitive conditioning we acquire throughout life.

It's very 'chicken and egg', as one issue seems to contribute to the other. For example, trauma changes the chemical balance of our brain, while those with a poor physical balance are much more sensitive to upsetting events.

Professionals of a more psychological orientation will say the psycho-social factors are the more important issue, while those of a more biological orientation will say the biology is the dominant issue. I don't think it can be so easily answered, or that these two issues can even be clearly divided. Clearly they are both important.

I'm sure the answer is highly individual. For example, if anxiety is caused by mercury toxicity, then mindfulness can only go so far. Whereas if stress is caused by a loved one's life being at risk or high levels of physical pain, then tinkering with brain chemistry can only go so far.

Stress seems to be a balance between the biological state, the psychological/cognitive factors and the external situation.

If the first two are in optimal balance then people are resilient to all but the more extreme stress.

The concept of 'total load' is a good way to think about it. Issues in each of the three categories can be thought of as additive and if they go beyond a certain threshold, tipping point, then stress will arise.

If imbalance rises high enough in one or more category then stress will be a problem.

What are some examples of how you have restored balance in the body and reduced negative stress?

One man I recall describing himself as 'burnt out from stress'. He suffered exhaustion, anxiety, depression, insomnia and was very emotionally reactive. As precipitating factors he cited a host of varied major life stressors. His lab tests confirmed he was burnt out.

Our normal stress hormone, cortisol, is secreted in above normal levels when initially under periods of stress.

Over time however levels become depleted. A normal morning saliva cortisol is around 25, which is associated with good energy, focus and stress resilience. This man's morning cortisol levels were 6. He also had signs suggestive of multiple neurochemical imbalances, presumably largely due to chronic stress.

He was treated with amino acids to raise neurotransmitter levels, B-vitamins, fish oil, an adrenal supporting supplement and melatonin for sleep. He wrote to me:

"I am feeling so much better than I did when we first consulted over 6 months ago. To give you an idea, for the last month I have been doing about 500 metres of swimming + 2 kms of walking about 5 times a week. This compares to struggling to do the weekly shopping! The feelings of exhaustion are not very common anymore. Depression and anxiety totally under control. Sleeping is much better. Overall, I am beginning to feel like a completely different person."

Another highly stressed woman I have worked with has ADHD (Attention Deficit Hyperactivity Disorder). We discovered she has very high needs for vitamin B6. After increasing her B6 a second time she wrote to me:

"I can't believe how much better I am in every way since increasing the B6 again. I can read easier, concentrate more, sleep through the entire night nearly always, I can dream and it is even in colour sometimes, more confident, I am more happy more often and catch myself laughing at times (usually MISS SERIOUS)."

How can we ride the waves of change in life around us without getting stressed? What practical steps do you recommend to help overcome stress?

There are various angles to address stress. The best results come from working in multiple areas.

Start by observing the basic requirements of health.

Eat an unrefined/nutrient dense diet, get 8-9 hours sleep/ night, avoid environmental exposures, do daily aerobic exercise, spend some time in the sun and nature, and include fun, rest, love and meaning in your life.

Investigate methods of addressing the thinking patterns and identification with these compulsive negative thoughts which contribute to stress.

For example study the books and DVD's of Eckhart Tolle, author of 'The Power of Now' and 'A New Earth'. He teaches methods of watching your mind rather than being controlled by your mind, accepting vs. resisting life's happenings, and experiencing the present moment rather than living constantly in the past or future.

Practice 30 minutes per day of some form of deep physiologic relaxation. This is very different than the kind of relaxation you get when sitting on the couch and watching TV.

I often recommend people choose one or more from the following list. This helps to train the body to be more relaxed generally and breaks the cycle of stress.

I personally use both the emwave biofeedback system and Holosync CD's for 30 minutes per day.

1. RelaxMate II photostimulation glasses designed by Dr. Norman Shealy. www.selfhealthsystems.com . Dr. Shealy's glasses produce pulses of coloured light at specific frequencies. Our brainwave pattern'follows'the emitted frequency enabling us to induce a state of deeper brain activity. Slow theta frequencies are generally most productive of deep relaxation. Published research has documented that photostimulation produces brain wave synchronization and increases levels of endorphins, serotonin and oxytocin. (Shealy. 1996) In one study all participants reported quick relaxation (most above 75%), 16/16 reported improved sleep, 12/12 reported reduced anxiety and 9/10 reported reduced depression. (Schmadel)

2. Guided imagery/meditation audio tracks. These CD's combine elements of progressive muscle relaxation, relaxing sounds/beats, guided imagery and hypnosis.
    *   Stress Management CD or MP3. www.mindmotivations.com
    *   Stress Relief Through Guided Imagery by Dr. Martin Rossman. www.thehealingmind.org
    *   Letting Go Of Stress by Dr. Emmett Miller. www.drmiller.com

3. Emwave stress relief technology by HeartMath. www.heartmath.com.au An innovative biofeedback system based on Heart Rate Variability, training you to reach a state of heart and mind coherence.

4. Holosync audio technology. www.meditate.com.au & www. centerpointe.com . Uses brain entraining audio technology placed beneath soothing music and listened to with stereo headphones. A free demo CD is available at these websites.

5. Meditation. Meditation can be learnt from classes, online programs or from books.

If your stress relates to past upsets and various conditioned reactions/ feelings (e.g. irritations to someone, compulsions, phobias, etc.) seek methods to address these.

My personal preference for this is what are termed either 'energy psychology' or 'neuro-physiological' techniques, which break patterns of conditioning and release emotional charge from past events. These include EFT (Emotional Freedom Techniques) (www.emofree.com.au), BMSA (Brief Multisensory Activation Therapy) (www.bmsa-int.com) and others.

These often achieve what traditional counselling never does. They are amazing for post-traumatic stress syndrome. I use them when I am upset about something and find it very effective.

See a practitioner of nutritional/environmental medicine who can help investigate and address a variety of biological health issues which may be contributing to your stress levels.

How can people find a health practitioner trained in nutrition and environmental medicine?

ACNEM provides a service to put members of the public in touch with medical doctors, dentists and other practitioners in Australia and New Zealand who have graduated from the ACNEM Primary Course. There are also some medical doctors and dentists on the referral list in other countries - Malaysia, Hong Kong and South Africa.

ACNEM (Australasian College of Nutritional and Environmental Medicine) www.acnem.org

Blake, what inspires you each day?

Love. The love I have for my partner in life, her eyes, her smile, her laugh and her touch.

Chapter 4: *Nutrition Healing - Vitamins, Minerals, Fatty Acids and Mental Health*

What are 3 things you are grateful for in your life?

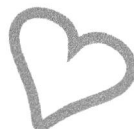

1. My beautiful woman.
2. The amazing gift of health.
3. The gift to help others.

I am truly blessed!

POWER ACTIONS FOR TODAY

Fun – do something today that you love and laugh. Laughter IS the best medicine.

Rest – Give yourself time out during the day.

- If you work at a computer or desk, get up every ½ hour and stretch your legs, pull your arms behind your back to open you chest up, take 3 FULL DEEP BREATHS, Let Go, Release, Relax as you breathe out.
- Create a 5-10 minute break in the day, every day, to refresh yourself.
- Set a time that you go home and don't work too late. Give yourself quality time out.
- Plan 8-9 hours sleep at night to allow your body to rest.

Love – Yourself and your fellow sentient beings.

Meaning – What's important to you? What gives you a sense of meaning to your life? What is your passion? What makes your heart sing? How can you nourish and nurture that in your life?

"When one door of happiness closes, another opens; but often we look so long at the closed door that we do not see the one which has been opened for us."

Helen Keller

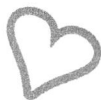

SIMPLE SELF-LOVE MEDITATION

Love begins with you.

Close your eyes and take a few long deep breaths.

You are able to feel the calm and stillness within you more easily each day.

As you let go of the outside world, begin to feel your spiritual connection to every living thing.

There is no separation, feel yourself in harmony with all that is.

Allow your mind to merge with the wind, the sun, the moon, the stars.

You are at peace with the harmony of nature all around you.

Continue breathing deeply and slowly.

Love has no restrictions. Love does not judge. Love dissolves hurt and anger.

Love is acceptance. I accept everyone, including myself, exactly as they are.

I accept and love myself. I am kind and gentle to myself.

Focus on your heart and with each deep breath, accept yourself with love.

The core of your being is love. Let love flow from your heart to touch those you love and all you come in contact with. Love heals all. Love can overcome all hurdles. Start with healing yourself. Listen to your heart, not your head.

Your mind is calm and still. Love is all there is.

Yes. Love is All There Is.

As you slowly and gently come out of Meditation, hold this feeling of love for yourself in your heart.

You will naturally be more loving to others as you grow this sense of love for yourself and all that is.

Go to www.HowToOvercomeStressNaturally.com/Resources
for an audio version of this meditation

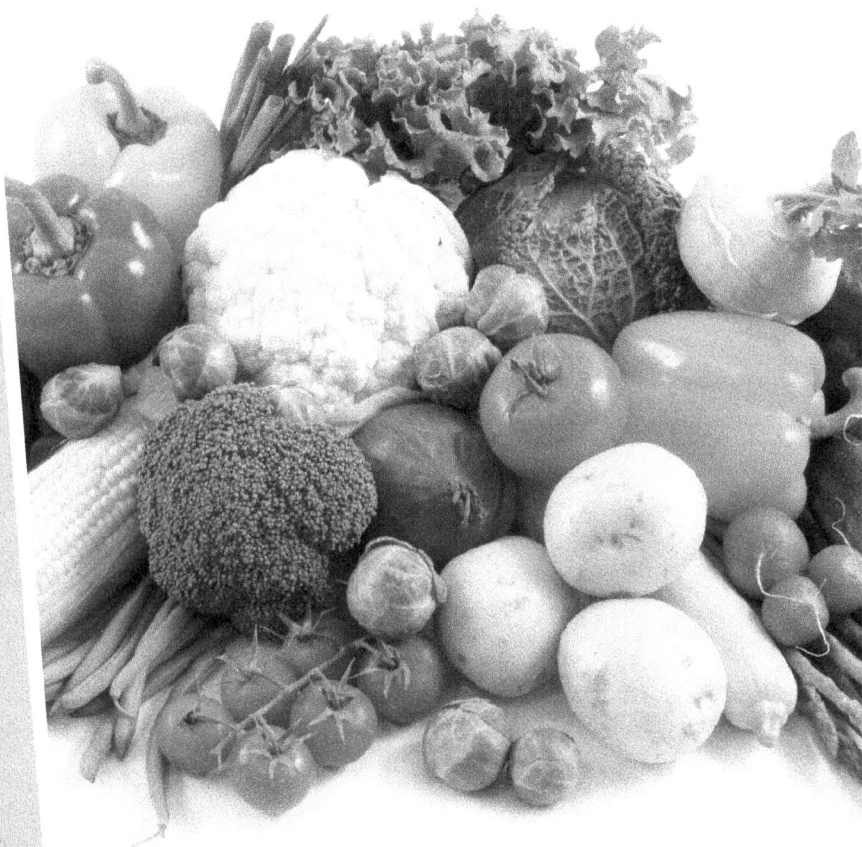

Chapter 5:

Change Your Food to Change Your Mood

Chapter 5:

Change Your Food to Change Your Mood

Julie Wood RN, GDHSc(NM), GDHSc(OH), Dip Aroma IAAMA 766, Dip Hyp Nutrition Medicine Practitioner & Aromatherapist

> A survey of 200 people in England reported that 88 percent found that changing their diet improved their mental health.
> *Survey conducted by the "Food and Mood Project", Amanda Geary, reported on BBC Health.*

I am a registered nurse, trained as a midwife and I have a passion for preventive medicine. I came from a school of nursing that was really interested in more preventive medicine than in treating disease, so we were always taught to look at ways of preventing disease. I then went into Family Planning and Occupational Health and worked in outback Australia setting up occupational health programs with some mining companies. I did post-graduate studies in occupational health and safety. I was one of the first nurses in Australia to do tertiary education at that level. I have University qualifications in Nutrition Medicine, Senior Clinical Tutor in the Master of Nutrition Medicine Program, at RMIT University.

My husband had a motorbike accident and was left with severe brain damage, so nutritiously the things that I did with him really saved his life and got him to the point where he is today. Independent, functioning, doing all the things that medically he wasn't supposed to do.

Let Julie share with you her vast knowledge on how to eat and improve your life enormously.

Foods and their Effect on Mood

Do you remember when you were a carefree, happy, energetic being who was relaxed and at one with the world? The world seemed simpler then and we were not rushing around between jobs, managing family, budgeting tightly, feeling "stressed" to the maximum and buying convenience foods to save time.

Chapter 5: *Change Your Food to Change Your Mood*

How many of us know the relationship between food and mood?

Brain Chemicals that Affect Your Mood

There are three main chemical neurotransmitters in the brain which help send messages from one cell to the next. They are dopamine, noradrenalin and serotonin.

- Dopamine and Noradrenalin are the brain chemicals that keep us alert: they have a tendency to make us think more quickly and they increase motivation, mental acuity and productivity.

- Serotonin on the other hand is the calming brain chemical: it produces a relaxed, more focused, less anxious, less stressed, more euphoric feeling.

Levels of these neurotransmitters are directly related to the foods we eat and the nutrients they contain.

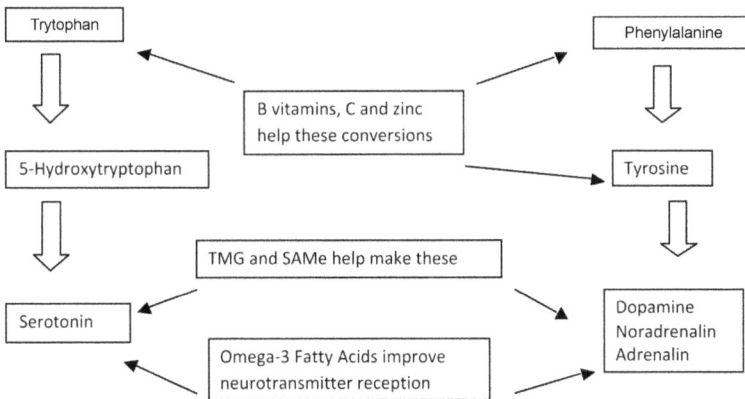

Trytophan		Phenylalanine
⬇	B vitamins, C and zinc help these conversions	⬇
5-Hydroxytryptophan		Tyrosine
⬇	TMG and SAMe help make these	⬇
Serotonin		Dopamine Noradrenalin Adrenalin
	Omega-3 Fatty Acids improve neurotransmitter reception	

CHANGE THE FOODS TO CHANGE YOUR MOOD

Isn't it nice to know that in many cases if you change the foods that you eat it can have a positive impact on your mood and change the chemical balance in the brain.

How does food affect mood?

There are many explanations for the cause-and-effect relationship between food and mood. The following are some examples:

- Fluctuations in blood sugar levels are associated with changes in mood and energy, and are affected by what we eat.
- Brain chemicals (neurotransmitters, such as serotonin, dopamine and acetylcholine) influence the way we think, feel and behave. They can be affected by what we've eaten.
- There can be abnormal reactions to artificial chemicals in foods, such as artificial colourings and flavourings.
- There are reactions that can be due to the deficiency of an enzyme needed to digest a food. Lactase, for instance, is needed to digest lactose (milk sugar). Without it, a milk intolerance can build up.
- People can become hypersensitive to foods. This can cause what are known as delayed or hidden food allergies or sensitivities.
- Low levels of vitamins, minerals and essential fatty acids can affect mental health, with some symptoms associated with particular nutritional deficiencies. For example, links have been demonstrated between low levels of certain B-vitamins and symptoms of schizophrenia, low levels of the mineral zinc and eating disorders, and low levels of omega-3 oils and depression.
- A build-up of toxins from the environment, such as lead from traffic pollution or mercury from leaky amalgam fillings, can also affect the proper functioning of the body and brain.
- Poor digestion leading to an accumulation of undigested foods in the gut can result in poor absorption of nutrients and a build up of toxins or malabsorption in the bowel leading to bowel dysbiosis "Leaky gut", our bowel has a large number of neurotransmitter receptors and these can be affected, as well as toxins escaping the bowel and ending up in the brain interfering with the neurotransmitters in the brain.

Chapter 5: *Change Your Food to Change Your Mood*

Choosing the Right Foods

Protein

- Incorporating the best quality foods into your daily life will help you stay on an even keel. Protein encourages the production of dopamine and noradrenalin, which produces alertness, mental energy and faster reaction time. The effects of eating protein last about 2 – 3 hours.

- If you have trouble sleeping make sure that you have your last protein meal several hours before you go to bed.

- **Fish** such as salmon, mackerel and sardines are rich in omega-3 fatty acid. Research has shown that omega-3 is used for building neurotransmitters like serotonin in the brain, helps reduce depression and also has anti-inflammatory properties.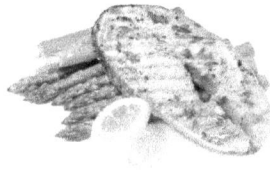

- **Sardines** are also high in zinc and calcium – with their bones.

- **Chicken and turkey** are also recognised as being higher in their levels of tryptophan which naturally boosts serotonin levels.

- **Lean red meat** also has small amounts of tryptophan and tyrosine – another amino acid our brain requires.

- **Oysters** are high in zinc as is crab.

Vegetables

- **Artichokes:** This odd-looking vegetable is fat-free, a good source of complex carbohydrates, and contains fructooligosaccharides (FOS), a non-digestible fibre. The human body does not possess the enzymes required to break down FOS. However, bacteria found in the large intestine and colon does contain the enzymes. For this reason, artichokes are beneficial to people who experience bowel problems. Artichokes are a good source of iron, potassium, magnesium, copper and manganese. They provide nearly 20 percent of the RDA for vitamin C, 23 percent of vitamin K and 17 percent folate. One artichoke contains around 76 calories.

- **Broccoli:** Research has proven broccoli has the potential to prevent cancer. That fact alone should make you want to eat it on a daily basis. Broccoli has also been proven effective in lowering the risk of heart disease and stroke. Broccoli is rich in beta carotene, calcium, iron, folate, vitamin C and E, and zinc. Broccoli contains about 15 percent of tryptophan; an essential amino acid that aids in sleep and relaxation. Eat this food throughout the day and for an evening snack to keep your nerves calm and to obtain a peaceful sleep.

- **Garlic:** One of the most notable benefits of garlic is its ability to reduce blood pressure. Garlic is also known for its antibacterial properties, which can reduce the risk of infection and illness. Recent studies show garlic may also help reduce the risk of heart disease and cancer.
  At only 9 calories per clove, it is a perfect vegetable for those watching their weight. Garlic is a good source of manganese, vitamin B6, vitamin C and calcium. Garlic can be eaten raw, added to nearly every recipe, or baked for a delicious garlic spread. Garlic salt or garlic powder can be used as a salt substitute.

- **Onions:** Not only are onions a good source of fibre, potassium, and B vitamins, they also possess anti-inflammatory and anti-cancer properties. Research indicates onions may help to reduce the risk of heart attack and stroke, and relieve bronchial congestion.
  At only 36 calories per medium-sized onion, these flavourful veggies can be abundantly consumed on a daily basis. Raw onions provide the highest level of health benefits. Add a splash of extra virgin olive oil to onion slices and toss on the grill. Fresh herbs and spices can be added for an extra punch of flavour. Add red onion to your salad.

- **Tomatoes:** Perhaps one of the most versatile vegetables (fruits) is the tomato. It can be eaten raw, cooked, steamed, grilled, baked, juiced, or pureed. Tomatoes are compatible with nearly every type of food including meats, vegetables, potatoes and rice. Tomato paste has the highest concentration of antioxidants and just a teaspoon a day will work for you.

They are a good source of vitamins C and E. Just one cup will provide you with more than 50 percent of the RDA of vitamin C, 20 percent of vitamin A and 15 percent of vitamin K. Tomatoes also contain lycopene, a phytochemical known to reduce the risk of heart disease.

- **Spinach:** Is a potent green. Part of the family that includes kale and chard, spinach is a rich source of several minerals that are good for anxiety and depression.

  Spinach contains magnesium, a mineral with relaxing and calming effects.

  Green leafy vegetables are also high in folic acid, low levels of which have been linked to depression in several studies. Other foods loaded with folic acid include sunflower seeds, green leafy vegetables, broccoli, wheat germ, oatmeal, black-eyed peas, lentils, soybeans and mustard greens.

- **Sweet potatoes:** Eating complex carbohydrates sets off a process that results in boosting your levels of serotonin. This brain chemical packs a wallop when it comes to mood enhancement. Carbs trigger the production of insulin, which clears glucose and amino acids from the bloodstream. This process paves the way for another amino acid, tryptophan, to cross the blood-brain barrier and get to work on boosting serotonin levels.

Complex carbs offer far more nutritional value than biscuits, candy and soft drink, and they're more slowly absorbed in your bloodstream, which contributes to keeping blood-sugar levels — and your mood — stabilized.

FRUITS:

- **Apricots:** These beauties are rich in the antioxidant beta carotene; the molecule that gives fruits and vegetables their orange colour. Apricots also contain an abundant supply of iron and potassium. They help regulate blood pressure and maintain regular bowel function. If you ever experience constipation, eat an apricot! One fresh apricot provides an adult with one-fifth of the daily recommended value of potassium. It also packs a whopping 20 percent of the RDA of vitamin A, 8 percent vitamin C, and 5 percent fibre. Apricots contain tryptophan, which helps to induce sleep and relaxation.

- **Avocados:** Oftentimes, people shy away from avocados because of their fat content. However, avocados contain "good" fat and are rich in vitamins C, E, and B6. They are also a good source of potassium. Studies have shown avocados possess the ability to reduce cholesterol. Individuals diagnosed with atherosclerosis (hardening of the arteries) can obtain benefits by consuming two to three avocados per week. Avocados are high in calories, so limit weekly consumption to a maximum of three.

- **Bananas:** Need a quick energy boost? Eat a banana. This delectable fruit contains only 62 calories and is rich in potassium and vitamin B6. It also boasts vitamin C and dietary fibre. Look for bananas which are not fully ripened because they contain less starch than fully ripened bananas.

Bananas are probably one of the most versatile health foods available. They can be eaten with every meal, as a snack or dessert. You can add them to frozen yogurt or a fruit salad. They can be grilled, broiled, sautéed or flambéed. A favourite banana recipe is to insert a popsicle stick into a banana, coat in melted dark chocolate, roll in chopped nuts and freeze. There's nothing better on a hot summer night!

- **Blueberries:** This tart berry has been shown to reduce inflammation; making blueberries a good choice for individuals with arthritis and other inflammatory diseases. Research shows that eating thirty blueberries per day can help alleviate aches and pains in the joints.

In addition to being an anti-inflammatory fruit, blueberries also offer anti-blood clotting and antibacterial effects. They can help ease the pain associated with diarrhoea or food poisoning. Blueberries contain the highest level of antioxidants and are said to possess anti-aging properties. One cup of blueberries contains less than 100 calories, yet provides nearly 30 percent of the RDA for vitamin C, 10 percent vitamin E, and 15 percent dietary fibre. They can be added to cereal, oatmeal, fruit salads, and yogurt or eaten plain. Add dried blueberries to muffin mix and eat as an afternoon snack .

Chapter 5: *Change Your Food to Change Your Mood*

- **Mangoes:** Mangoes contain beta-cryptoxanthin, a potent antioxidant that prevents free radicals from damaging your cells and DNA. Recent studies have shown that mangoes may help to reduce the risk of colon and cervical cancer. Mangoes are rich in beta carotene, which is converted to vitamin A within the body. It's important to note that beta-cryptoxanthin is best absorbed by the body when eaten with fat. For best results, consume mangoes as part of a meal.

Mango salsa makes an excellent companion with chicken and pork. They add a tart, yet sweet flavour to fruit salads and smoothies. Mangoes can be frozen, but be certain to remove the skin and core and store in a freezer bag.

Nuts and Seeds

- **Pumpkin Seeds:** Pumpkin seeds are a good source of magnesium. Magnesium plays an important role in heart health and helps strengthen bones and teeth. It also helps the body absorb key minerals such as calcium and potassium. A glaring symptom of magnesium deficiency is depression (in addition to loss of appetite, leg cramps and migraines). This can be attributed to magnesium's role in serotonin production (see above for a more detailed discussion of the mood-boosting benefits of serotonin). Other sources of magnesium include halibut, quinoa, chia, spinach, plums and tomatoes.

- **Sunflower Seeds:** One of the most popular seeds consumed, sunflower seeds are rich in vitamin E and known to reduce the risk of heart disease and cancer. Studies have also shown them effective in guarding against cataracts. Experts recommend eating two tablespoons of sunflower seeds each day. Doing so will double your intake of vitamin E. However, they are high in calories and should be eaten in limited quantities.

- **Chia Seeds:** New kid on the block to us but known to the Aztecs for hundreds of years. The seeds are high in protein, magnesium, potassium, phosphorous and have the highest level of omega-3 known. This amazing little seed is taken daily – 1 dessert spoon soaked in water.

- **Almonds:** Classified as a nut, almonds are actually the seed of the fruit of an almond tree. They offer a delicate and mild flavour to dishes and can be added to vegetables, meats, fruits and desserts. Eating twelve almonds per day can provide you with the recommended daily allowance of essential fatty acids. Almonds are rich in potassium and are considered a "good" fat. These fruit seeds are high in calories, so limit your intake to no more than twelve per day. They should be lightly roasted or sprouted. Use almond meal in cake mixes and muffins.

- **Brazil nuts:** Brazil nuts contain all the essential amino acids, making them a complete protein. Brazil nuts contain exceptionally high levels of selenium; a powerful antioxidant that can help reduce the risk of heart disease and cancer.

Brazil nuts are an excellent source of zinc, which is essential to digestion and metabolism. Brazil nuts contain a high level of fat and should not be consumed more than three times per week. One serving equals eight nuts and is equivalent to 30 grams of fat.

Don't Forget the Spices

- **Black Pepper:** Either purchase a peppermill and fill it with black peppercorns, white peppercorns or red peppercorns, or a mixture. Freshly ground pepper adds zest to any dish, especially lean steaks and roasts. Pepper is one of the world's healthiest spices because it is known for its positive effect on the digestive tract. It also has antibacterial and antioxidant benefits. Pepper also provides Vitamin A, Calcium, Copper, Vitamin K, Iron, Manganese, Magnesium and Potassium.

- **Cayenne Pepper:** is derived from hot chili peppers. Cayenne pepper is great at fighting inflammation. Cayenne pepper is rich in Vitamin A, and also provides Iron, Manganese, Niacin, Niacin, Magnesium and Potassium, Riboflavin, Vitamin A, Vitamin C, Vitamin E, Vitamin K and Vitamin B6, making it one of the world's healthiest spices.

Chapter 5: *Change Your Food to Change Your Mood*

- **Chili Pepper:** Dried chili pepper powder adds heat and spice to chili, hot wings, and ethnic foods. Similar to cayenne pepper ground chili pepper provides anti-inflammatory benefits, as it contains capsaicin. Dried chili pepper is one of the world's healthiest spices because it is also a good source of Vitamin A, Vitamin C, Potassium, Iron and dietary fibre.

- **Cinnamon:** If you cringe when you think of cinnamon, because the ground cinnamon you've tasted is bitter, try using Chinese Cinnamon. Chinese Cinnamon is sweeter, and has no bitter flavour. For a healthy snack, or fruit dip, combine equal parts non-fat vanilla or plain yogurt with unsweetened applesauce. Add cinnamon, and you have a healthy and nutritious snack.

  Ground cinnamon is not only very low in cholesterol, and in sodium, it is low in saturated fat. Cinnamon also boosts your vitamin intake with its Vitamin C , Iron, Manganese, and Vitamin K. In addition to exuding an incredible aroma when cooked, cinnamon has health-promoting properties, making it one of the world's healthiest spices. Cinnamon promotes anti-clotting, can control blood sugar and improves digestive health. Ideal to add to your black coffee instead of sugar , 1/8th teaspoon a day is all you need.

- **Cloves:** One of those spices that an unseasoned cook may not use much. For ham eaters, the little unopened flower bud twigs are a familiar site. Cloves can also be used in Swedish meatballs, with dishes using beans, and in delicious desserts like molasses cookies, pumpkin pie, gingerbread and ginger snaps.

  One of the world's healthiest spices, cloves add Beta Cryptoxanthin, Calcium, Magnesium, Potassium Vitamin A and Vitamin C to your food. Cloves can be used to treat digestive tract cancers. Cloves also offer anesthetic and anti-bacterial qualities and are used in oral care products, as well as in substances used by dentists.

- **Ginger:** Because ginger is a root, it is considered a spice and not an herb. Ginger can be added to chicken, beef or vegetable dishes, as well as desserts like Gingerbread.

Ginger, like most spices, is low in cholesterol, low in saturated fat, and low in sodium. Ginger is one of the world's healthiest spices and provides Copper, Manganese, Magnesium, Potassium, and Vitamin C. Ginger, even when used in Ginger Ale, is known for its positive effects on an upset stomach, or medically, on gastrointestinal distress. Ginger is a great way to quell motion sickness. It also has some anti-inflammatory benefits.

- **Mustard Seeds:** refers to actual mustard seeds, or ground mustard, not that bright yellow concoction in the familiar pull-top bottle. Mustard adds depth to any chicken dish, or cold potato salad. Mustard can also be used with a vinaigrette to make a delicious cold or warm dressing. Mustard seeds are one of the world's healthiest spices because they are a good sources of calcium, iron, magnesium, phosphorus and protein, as well as Lutein and Zeaxanthin. They also boast Omega 3 fatty acids. Mustard seeds are also a great source of selenium. Selenium is considered to have cancer-prevention qualities, anti-inflammatory qualities, and can even lessen the severity of asthma.

- **Tumeric:** A popular ingredient in curry powder, Tumeric is part of the Ginger family, and another one of the world's healthiest spices. Tumeric is tasty when cooked with lentils and other vegetarian dishes. Tumeric is low in cholesterol and low in sodium. The yellow tumeric also provides dietary fibre, Iron, Manganese, Magnesium, Vitamin B6, Vitamin C, and Potassium. Tumeric is considered one of the world's healthiest spices because of its anti-inflammatory qualities, it aids in digestion and it can help heal wounds.

Chapter 5: *Change Your Food to Change Your Mood*

Some Tips

ANGRY?	DEPRESSED?	Need to be more **MENTALLY ALERT?**
Eat a grapefruit! It's rich in pectin, a soluble fibre that lowers blood cholesterol and reverses the negative effects anger has on the body. Grapefruit also contains vitamin C, potassium, calcium and iron.	Try a bowl of plain rice, a low-fat, no-cholesterol complex carbohydrate full of selenium, which may ward off depression.	Reach for an apple. It contains lots of boron, which helps boost mental alertness.
CHOCOLATE ANYONE?	**TIRED AND DEPRESSED?**	**FEELING OLD?**
Cocoa contains phenylethylkamine -- a compound that is released in the brain when emotionally aroused (many say the effects resemble the feeling of falling in love). Chocolate also contains phenols, antioxidants that reduce heart disease.	Grab a handful of raisins, rich in iron.	Fill up on carrots, an excellent source of beta-carotene, which is not only famous for promoting healthy eyesight, but decelerates the aging process.

Aromatherapists also have access to a myriad of oils that provide a precise blend of chemicals that can affect mood and behaviour.

For example:
Mood Booster – Neroli, Bergamot, Rose Geranium, Petigrain
Relaxant – Lavender, Lemon, Marjoram, Sandalwood

How about making some Peppermint Chia Balls

What you will need is:

~ 450gm tahina

~ Either 1 cup organic cocoa with ¾ cup Agave

~ Or 1 cup Carob with ¾ cup honey

~ ½ - ¾ cup coconut flour

~ 100gm chia seeds – ground to a flour

~ 10 drops peppermint essential oil

What you will need to do:

Mix well and roll into small balls and refrigerate.

How Many?

100 balls = 10gm/ball   50 balls = 20gm/ball

Optional

Can add figs/ prunes or nut meal as well or use a different essential oils such as orange, and perhaps some drops of rose water.

Julie, what, in your experience, is the fundamental root cause of stress that will reflect in our bodies?

We all need a certain level of stress. Otherwise we wouldn't function. Stress is a normal psychological reaction. We have stress when we eat, because that puts stress on the nervous-system to produce the right enzymes to break down the food. So we have some level of stress all the time.

It's the chronic, ongoing stress that causes the problem. Like being a full time carer, or like being in a violent relationship. Or like working sixteen hours a day for poor pay or being put in situations where we are constantly under stress, and we have that fight/flight cortisol mechanism that we have in our body, but we've got nowhere to go with it.

That affects a whole range of things in our body, our anabolic hormones and cortisol levels get affected which then suppresses our digestive functions. Then we don't eat properly because we are not hungry or we get indigestion.

What do you recommend as the 1st step to overcome stress naturally?

1. I look at changing the diet, just the simple things.
2. Just take ten minutes and sit down and eat lunch. Take the time to do that.
3. Meditation is something I always suggest.
4. Walk, if they can. Go for a walk, along the river, down the beach, even if it's just around the shopping centre.
5. Go and have a coffee with somebody, and simply have a chat.
6. Aromatherapy. Burn some aromatherapy oils or have a massage, a foot massage. It starts to lift the spirit.
7. Make the stressful situation a challenge. Look at how we can get out of it, or change it, or what we can do rather than being a victim in it.

Chapter 5: *Change Your Food to Change Your Mood*

I have clients say all and every day, "If you had told me two months ago, that just changing my diet would affect my mood, I would have told you to get lost. That it was silly or wouldn't happen."

Initially it was difficult to change what they are eating, but after they had done it for a couple of weeks, they could see the light; suddenly there's a light at the end of the tunnel, where there was nothing there before.

Their depression was so great that they couldn't do anything and they just cried all day, and suddenly when we change what they're eating, it's suddenly impacting on how they're feeling.

The analogy is with the fuel you put in your car. If you put the wrong fuel in your car it's not going to run very well, or it's going to break down more often. It's the same with our body. What fuel we put in and how it is broken down determines how well we function. We need nutrients to drive the energy in our cells.

Coffee, Cake & Chocolate

I have all my clients on coffee. It must be black coffee, because it is a good antioxidant.

Use cinnamon, instead of sugar. It's much better. Also cinnamon is an antioxidant that helps stabilize your blood sugar level.

I also give my clients Dark chocolate - because there are antioxidants in it.

Have Your Cake and Eat It Too - Make muffins that are high in protein and high in fibre!

We all have to look for new ways. Especially today when it's such a time of change. It's a great place to Start; taking care of ourselves, and being healthy and eating the right food.

Yes. Definitely. That's going to become more and more important because we're so exposed to toxins everyday. We need to be able to have some diet or eating that helps our body to detoxify.

Food is so important. It's amazing. I love to see how it changes people. The whole family benefits.

In America there are some specialists and programs that now specialise in treating genetic problems with high dose nutrition. The focus is on food and nutrients. They can change DNA or RNA patterns.

Where can people find you Julie?

I have my clinic at Runaway Bay, Gold Coast, Queensland.
Website: **www.naturallyhealthy.com.au**

What are three things that you are grateful for?

1. I am grateful for being given so many opportunities to learn- I've had some amazing teachers. I'm really grateful to them for taking me and allowing me to work with them, because they've taught me things that normally people wouldn't be exposed to, you know.
2. I'm grateful in some ways that my husband had his accident, because it really enabled me to move into an area that I really wanted to go into, even though it's been very traumatic. We all go through some depression at some point. But it's how we deal with it.
3. And I'm really grateful that I'm able to share my knowledge with other people. So I am grateful for being alive.

Chapter 5: *Change Your Food to Change Your Mood*

References

1. Vitetta L, Anton B, Cortizo F, Sali A. Mind-body medicine: Stress and its impact on overall health and longevity. Ann NY Acad Sc. 2005: 1057:492-505

2. Young E et al. Psychoneuroendocrinology of depression: hypothalamic-pituitary-gonadal axis. In: Nemeroff CB (ed) Psychoneuroendocrinology The Psychiatric Clin of Nth Amer 1998. 21, 309-324

3. Leonard B. Stress, depression and the activation of the immune system. World J Biol Psychiatry. 2000; 1(1): 17-25 Review

4. Coppen A, Bolander-Gouaille C. Treatment of depression: time to consider folic acid and vitamin B12. J Psychopharmacol. 2005 Jan; 19(1): 59-65

5. Hvas AM et al. Vitamin B6 level is associated with symptoms of depression. Psychother Psychosom. 2004 Nov-Dec; 73(6):340-343

6. Beard JL et al. Maternal iron deficiency anaemia affects postpartum emotions and cognition. J Nutr. 2005 Feb; 135(2): 267-72

7. International Summit For Mental Health – Transcripts and References. 2006, 2007, 2008

8. Pfeiffer Treatment Centre: http://www.hriptc.org/index.php in USA

9. Australian contact for Pfeiffer Protocols: Bio-Balance Health: http://www.biobalance.org.au/

10. Sydney-Smith M: Course Material: Master of Nutrition Medicine program. Australian College of Holistic Medicine. RMIT University. www.nutritionmedicine.org

3 PRACTICAL HEALTHY TIPS FOR TODAY
Love & Respect your body

1. Start Your Day with Protein – Have some salmon or sardines to boost alertness and faster reaction time. (Protein encourages production of dopamine and noradrenaline.)

REMEMBER: The effects of eating protein last about 2-3 hours.

2. Eat an Apple today – to boost your mental alertness.

3. Feeling tired? – Eat some raisons which are rich in iron.

MINDFULNESS – FOOD PRAYER – GIVE THANKS

Be aware and grateful of the food you put into your body every day. Fuel for your temple. The body that carries you around day after day.

I give thanks for the food we are about to eat that gives us nourishment.
I prepare this food with love.

Here is a simple prayer:
Thank you for the world so sweet,
Thank you for the food we eat,
Thank you for the birds that sing,
Thank you God for everything. Amen.

Make up your own heartfelt prayer of thanks for the food that nourishes you each day.

Take a moment to be Mindful before you eat, to give thanks and truly be grateful.

Respect and love yourself. Take the time to eat well EVERY day.

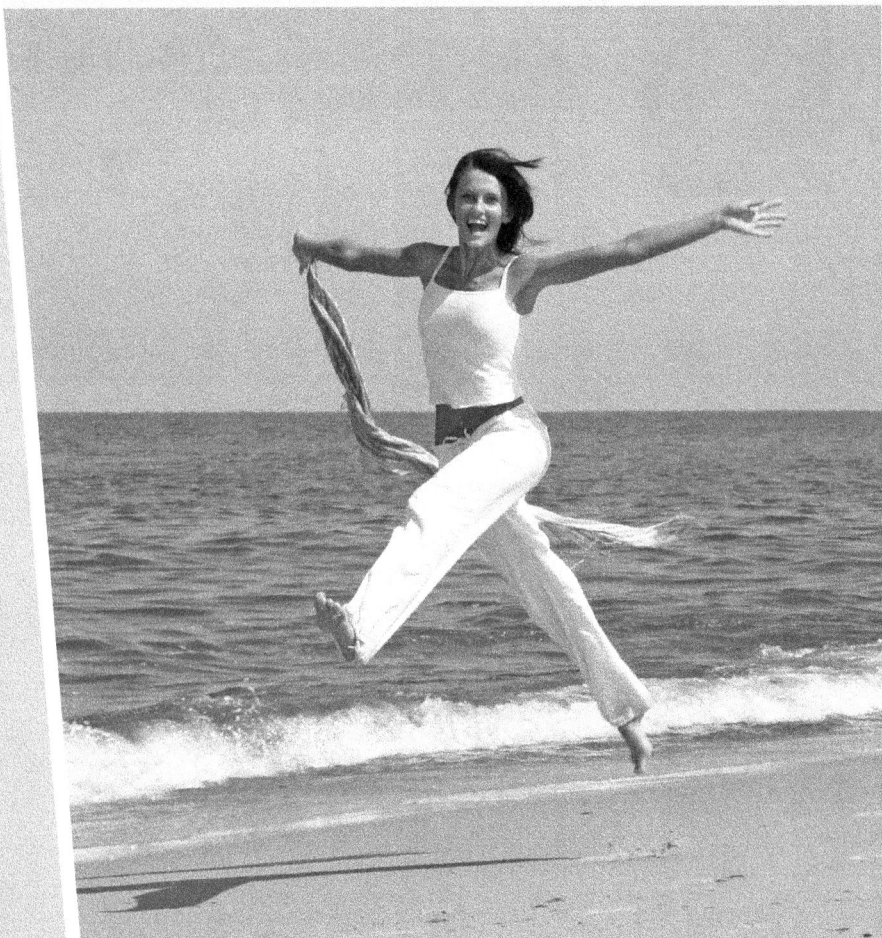

Chapter 6:

A New Way of Looking at Life – The Australian Depression Institute

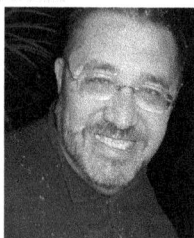

Chapter 6:

A New Way of Looking at Life – The Australian Depression Institute

Wayne Parrott: Founder Australian Depression Institute, Maleny, Queensland in conjunction with Fountainhead Organic Health Retreat, Maleny

Wayne, tell us how the Australian Depression Institute came to be and where it is today.

About 10 years ago my best friend was struck down with depression. After trying all the usual avenues he was still very sick.

I contacted Beyond Blue, the national depression initiative in Australia, and asked for advice. They gave me a number of names of therapies and a few people that they had heard good things about. I investigated all of these therapies and these people and I realised that mostly they were looking at parts of the problem. Very few seemed to confer with each other. They did not seem to share information with each other. What I decided to do was to take the best of each therapy and see if there was a method or a system that could work for most people.

I then tested this with over 3,000 clients at the Fountainhead Organic Health Retreat in Queensland. Over the ensuing 8 years I continued to search for additional therapies "that work". The fact that I have a non–medical background has enabled me to look for what worked only. I do not get caught in the jargon. I look from my client's point of view only.

What is the Australian Depression Institute Method?

In a retreat environment, (where this method was developed) you need to be able to take a lot of time away from home, (normally 28 days) for the program the Fountainhead Team uses.

Chapter 6: *A New Way of Looking at Life*
– The Australian Depression Institute

Obviously there are large costs involved with accommodation and food for this amount of time, plus the therapy cost. I formed the Australian Depression Institute, for those that were time poor and had a lower budget. We commenced business after a year of testing, only last October, 2008.

Now we can offer a solution that is very effective, that is available and affordable to all Australians. Even a single parent with a social welfare income could trade their life skills in some area to complete the course. If you're serious about doing something about depression, there are no more excuses. We have something for everyone.

What role does Fountainhead Holistic Health Retreat play?

It was where we developed and tested the "method". It continues to serve over 100 guests most months and has a cure rate claimed by the guests that is probably the highest in the world. The Life Coach team at Fountainhead save lives, every month. Greg Neville, a Naturopath, still lectures with us each month. Many Australian Depression Institute programs run from Fountainhead as their base. It will always be the spiritual centre.

Tell me a bit about Fountainhead Health Retreat.

We opened 7 years ago. It is now the only Certified Organic Retreat in the world. It's in a beautiful part of the world called Maleny, just near the Glass House Mountains in the Hinterland, Queensland.
Greg Neville is a Naturopath, who has been working with people with depression for years; Michelle Mark who has a Training background, developed the method into modules; and Salima Speranza, an experienced Life Coach, have been the key people in developing this Method.

Greg had already worked out a lot of this when we met and the girls have now turned the message into an easy to deliver, highly retained educational process. The other key developers have been the over 3,000 clients whom shared their life stories with us along the way. They were the real developers of this method because they showed us what really worked.

Do you use any prescription medicine at ADI?

If clients are on medication for their condition, we say stay on the medication. Medication can only be prescribed or told to stop being used by a doctor. We believe that is a good system that's already in place. Often the medication can be protecting the person from self harm or the depths of despair. Until the Method is clear in your Mind, it will not start to work. Come and get the message, get the information. Go back to your doctor. Only with doctor's advice and supervision can you wean yourself off.

In your opinion, what is the fundamental root cause of stress?

Life not going to plan, and our reactions to this perceived event. The reaction is often a fear; a self esteem doubt about our ability to deal with and learn from this reality.

There are external triggers but why does one person respond one way and someone else another way? i.e. I lost my job and I said to myself, "Oh it's time for a change. What do I want to do next?" Immediately I am in control of the situation rather than "It happened to me".

Very true. The person who looks for the lessons continues to make new plans and goals and accepts that maybe life was not meant to go to plan.

The depressed person however does something completely different. They will continue to look backward at the event; constantly re-living it, with lots of"what if's". This stops them moving forward. This damages their self esteem. Prevents the learning attached to the original event.

Can you explain how by addressing the core beliefs, there is a change in physical and emotional symptoms?

Certainly. Though Serotonin deficiency is still only just a theory, lets accept it as true and see if this method we have developed holds water if that is the case. And self esteem gets lower. The person whom develops depression has decided not to look forward. What is the good of planning ahead if these plans tend not to come to fruition? This thought process reduces new motor neuron pathway growth, and would contribute to this imbalance. Person number two; same event, different attitude, has no change in his brain chemicals and hence no imbalances are created.

In other words at Fountainhead we say "We are what we think".

Can you help if someone has a hormonal imbalance?

With over 3,000 people who were depressed already treated successfully at Fountainhead, we do not find the Method we use fails for simple depression or anxiety disorders. Other types of Depression have many multi layered psychological issues, sourced from past events, and then this is a different question. I think this is when you need a professional psychologist. For simple depression and anxiety this Method is very strong.

Can you help if someone has chemical imbalances in the brain?

Though as I mentioned it is still only theory, with the current evidence available, I would accept that all those depressed do in fact have some chemical imbalance in the brain. By treating the belief, you remedy this imbalance. That is why our system is so effective.

What if someone says "I can't change my life circumstances".

Very often this situation is true. But you may not need to think this way. You just need to change how you look at your "tough" circumstance.

> **You can't change the circumstance but you can change how you look at it.**

Can you give some examples of people who have come through the ADI programme?

Yes. Ian, a business person, had been sick for a long period time, approx 18 yrs, and been in mental hospitals and electrotherapy. I picked him up from the airport on the way to Fountainhead Retreat. He was very distant, we didn't really connect and he looked out the window a lot.

I went off to Melbourne for a conference and returned 2 weeks later. I was on a morning walk at Fountainhead when a man said "Hi" and I said "Hi" and he thanked me.

I said "Do I know you?" He said, "Wayne, you picked me up from the airport 2 weeks ago, it's Ian."

I said, "Ian, you look completely different."

His physical appearance had changed so much. I said "Well what do you think?"

"Wayne I'm embarrassed, it was so easy to learn," he said.

I said, "Nothing's easy and nothing's hard. It's only easy when you know how."

It's now 4 years since that meeting and Ian was back with his wife to visit us just a month ago.
In his own life he now helps others and shares his experience.

A lot of people who come through Fountainhead love to share their experience. We have treated 3 generations of one family. We sometimes follow clients home and help family members understand what the person has been educated on.

We have people as young as 14-15yr old come to the retreat, with parental guidance.

In your opinion, what is the 1st step on the path to overcoming daily stress?

1. Accept that we are here on earth to learn lessons in life and to share them with each other.
2. Understand the fact that if life does not go to plan, it is not bad news, it is the system that exists to make us grow.
3. It truly is a wonderful world.

What practical steps can you recommend to overcome stress?

Fountainhead gets 20,000 visits or enquiries per month from all over the world on the website, seeking information.

- Educate yourself;
- Get some education in stress management.

Chapter 6: *A New Way of Looking at Life – The Australian Depression Institute*

How can people find the Australian Depression Institute & Fountainhead Organic Health Retreat?

It's a great reason to visit the beautiful Sunshine Coast!
We will be expanding nationally over the next two years.
If you live in another state, you can call us to find out when we will be in your state.
We can also come to your businesses when there are a group of 8 people or more.

Ph: (61) 07 5494 2900
Web: http://adi.net.au/ http://www.fountainhead.com.au/

How can we ride the waves of change in life around us without getting stressed?

Accept that these upheavals are the very essence of life. Plenty of time after life to have less waves.

What is your strategy to deal with negative thoughts?

We do not believe in "negative and positive" thoughts. We teach accurate and inaccurate thoughts. Inaccurate understandings are what cause your stress. It's not so much the positive and negative. We see lots of positive people who are ill, and negative people who are well. It's about the accuracy and inaccuracy according to reality.

What keeps you personally motivated and focussed on a daily basis?

Understanding that the goal of my life is to learn and to teach others.

Is there anything else that is important for overcoming stress naturally?

If I was giving the advice to my 11 yr old daughter, I'd keep it simple.
- Accept that you are not on the wrong path. You can never be on the wrong path.
- Understand that you are having the exact life that you were meant to have to learn what you need to learn.
- Focus on the learning and your life will be a joy.

How does your 11 yr old respond?

My daughter grew up on a retreat, her mother is an artist / philosopher and her step-mother is a philosopher / trainer. So she is used to us talking a lot this way.

Who would you like to thank for helping develop your method?

My partner in life Michelle Mark whom now trains life coaches in this method, which without the ADI's creation would not have been possible.

Open minded passionate healers like Prof Bruno Cayoun, a top expert from Tasmania on Mindfulness, whom is teaching the team how to apply Mindfulness training, and examine some other traditional psychotherapies to see if they can improve our method further.

This is the attitude needed for us to create true holistic healing. Sharing, listening, and measuring.

Our only goal is the eradication of such illnesses.

What are 3 things you are grateful for in your life?

1. My life itself; that I am alive.
2. The love I have to give.
3. The ones in my life whom can accept this love.

I am surrounded by 46 staff and their ability to work with guests, their ability to give of themselves as they work toward solutions. It's an exciting world to work in.

3 PRACTICAL HEALTHY TIPS FOR TODAY

Listening – Be still Inside and Listen to a friend or stranger in need. Talk and share and listen.

Sharing – Phone a friend, talk to your dog, horse or cat, share your time with someone you enjoy.

Learning – Be Open to learn new ideas, new beliefs, new ways of thinking, living and being.

"Attitude is a little thing that makes a big difference."
Winston Churchill

CELEBRATE TODAY

Look for the joy in your life. Remember Life
is a Celebration. Lighten Up.
Delight in the wonder of every day.
Laugh and have Fun.
Relax and find your sense of humour.
See the good in others and share the joy of
life.
Play your favourite music and dance.
Angels fly because they take themselves
lightly. You can too.

"Always Look on the Bright Side of Life."
Monty Python

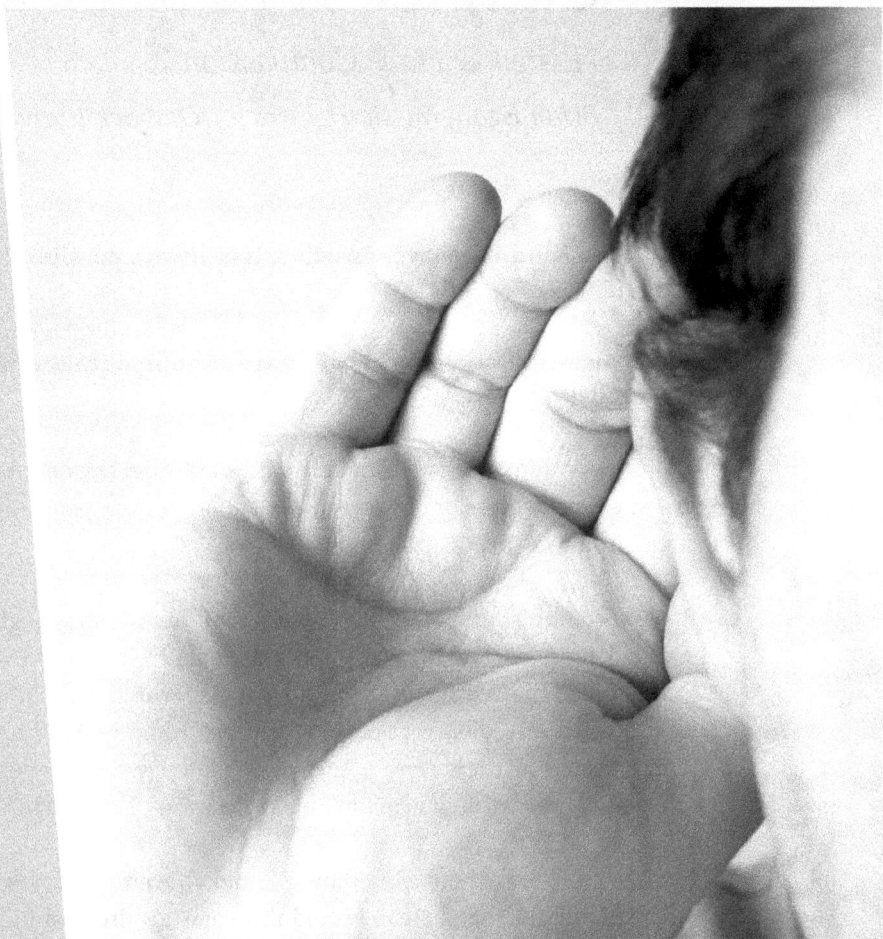

Chapter 7:

"Listen & Have Compassion"

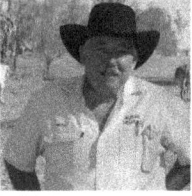

Chapter 7:

"Listen & Have Compassion"

Brian Egan. Aussie Helpers for Outback Farmers

"Be Kind Whenever Possible. It is always possible."
Dalai Lama

Brian, please tell us your background and your journey down the road of depression?

Well Trace, I think mine was an unusual sort of case, because it wasn't just stress or depression. I was actually suffering from post-traumatic stress, from war-related problems.

It was a combination of that, and losing our farm, which brought on a severe depression, and my whole life just seemed to be taken over by a thing I called the beast. This thing did just take over my thinking. That was quite an incredible sort of thing because I'd find myself having a panic, just sitting there crying. And I didn't know what was going on, or couldn't do anything. I couldn't make decisions, I couldn't.

I got to the stage where, you know, I couldn't even speak; I couldn't talk to people. By that, I mean I couldn't form words in my mind to get them out of my head; I think the doctors called it catatonic.

Combined with that I lost the ability to write. I can only write about one sentence at a time, and then my writing just goes berserk, as if some sort of entity has taken over my thinking and just squiggles away, so I use computers most of the time these days.

It was a horrible journey, and it lasted for about three years. I thank Veteran's Affairs for looking after me during that time, because otherwise, you know, I wouldn't be here today.

Chapter 7: *"Listen & Have Compassion"*

So as much as you were aware what was going on, there wasn't a way you could take control of the situation?

No, I started off with a G.P. like everybody else does. And, you know, you get your handout of Zoloft, or whatever it is, and they say it'll fix you up in six weeks, and off you go…and you still don't know what's wrong with you. You've got this thing controlling your mind, and you're taking these things, these anti-depressants. God knows what the difference is from anti-depressants and other psychotic sort of drugs, there must have been over twenty of them and all I got was severe side effects, shaking, sweating, hallucinations and stuff like that, which made life pretty well unbearable.

I really think that those sorts of things were probably the trigger to me trying to commit suicide twice. By then I'd just given up complete hope, and I couldn't see any future at all. I just called myself a gibbering idiot. That's what I was.

That's a long time, three years, Brian.

I was in hospital for over a year. Even The Head of Psychiatry at Greenslopes Hospital said something when they did Australian Story I was in. He said that they'd just given up on me; they didn't have much hope for me at all. But somehow, I've sort of come out of it.

I think there was a lot of help from another psychologist—who was actually a priest in another life. He'd fallen in love, and got married, and had kids, and so had become a psychologist.

He said to me one day: "Brian, your mind is that strong, I don't think drugs are ever going to fix your problem. I recommend that you go out and find somebody worse off than you are, and help them."

I just laughed at him. I said, "I've just walked off my farm. I've got absolutely nothing." I was fifty-five, or fifty-six, so I said, "I haven't got two bob to rub together. I haven't even got a house. I've got nothing." And he said, "Well, you'll find someone."

I was thinking of his previous life in the church, I think that he believed in miracles. He tragically got killed not long after that in an accident. But two years later I started up Aussie Helpers. I said, "His miracle did come true."

Would you say that was a turning point for you?

That was a turning point for me, yeah. He sort of really pushed me into doing something. When I left Greenslopes Hospital, they gave me a letter to take around to different charity organizations that said, 'Can you give this man some volunteer work because he's just out of hospital, etc., and he needs to face life in the community', because I wouldn't talk to anyone.

I started off just mowing lawns for people in this little country community. I used to do it for nothing, just to do something and because it was physical. These people would then talk to me, and I'd obviously answer them back, so I was communicating. That started it. Then I went and volunteered for the Salvation Army. I did that for a year or so, I went home one day to Nerida (my wife) and said, "Bugger this; I'm going to start my own charity." I still wasn't real flash then, but I just had this drive to get out and do something.

> I suppose there's been a bit of luck involved. But there's also been a passion to help other people too.

Tell me a bit about your charity - Aussie Helpers.

Aussie Helpers was a success that was born out of adversity. It was just a dream, a vision. Going back to that psychologist saying to go out and help somebody worse off than you. I thought, "Jeez, there's plenty of farmers that could do with a hand up, I can tell you". And that's how it started.

We never had any money. The whole organization started off with twenty dollars. We took food out of our own kitchen to make into a raffle, and the twenty dollars was used to buy raffle books. We started doing raffles in the pub. And that's how it kicked off.

Last financial year we received over a million dollars in donations from all over the place.

Chapter 7: *"Listen & Have Compassion"*

Fantastic.

It's just grown and grown, and keeps on growing.

It starts with one little step.

It does. And we've got sixteen vehicles on the road, and a couple of buildings; we don't have any debt. Because it's been so successful I think a lot of businesses and ordinary people get behind it, because they can see that we're just practical people, and we are actually doing what we say we do.

What do you actually do when you go out into the bush?

Well, it all started off with just me doing it, and I started off by going out and seeing schools around the Darling Downs area. It was way back in 2002 when the drought was pretty severe there. Kids were going to school without having brekkie, or any lunch, and I got on side with Kellogg's in Brisbane, and they donated all their seconds- sort of breakfast bars and muesli bars and stuff like that- tens of thousands of the things; then we got poppers from Golden Circle. We went out and gave cartons and cartons and cartons to different schools.

Within about a month or six weeks we had nearly fifty schools ringing up and asking us to come and see them, that's how bad the situation was. It was then we thought, "well, gee, if these kids are going to school without anything, there must not be anything at home". And so we started going out to the farms then, and taking out boxes of groceries and personal hygiene goods and stuff like that.

Does that continue to this day?

It does. Except we've just expanded a lot and it's not just me that does it now; there's probably about forty volunteers. We only have about six that actually do that on the road, because a lot of the time you come across people who need to talk to someone, which we call our face-to-face counselling, and it's sitting at a kitchen table at a farmhouse. We may just have a talk over a cup of tea.

> **People do open up. There are lots of hugs and tears and stuff like that. They just want somebody to listen, really.**

When I talk to my friends, when there's something I need to get off my chest, I often find a solution just in talking.

That's right. That's why we do that, because often these people do come up with their own solutions after we keep them talking about it.

The secret is just to sit down and listen to people.

You don't have to be a highly educated person with fifteen degrees after your name to be able to counsel someone, because ninety-nine percent of it's just listening.

Have a lot of compassion, or a bit of compassion for people.

Give people a hug that's what they need.

We are not out to save the world, I can tell you that, Tracey. But if we can help a few people it's what it's all about.

When you feel panicked or stressed these days what do you do?

I don't get stressed about anything anymore. I don't even worry anymore. I don't know why it's happened. People say you must get burnt out, or ask, "how do you debrief yourself after talking to so many people?" I just don't ever need to do it.

- I don't keep things in, for one thing.
- I just let it slide through, and off to see the next one.
- I don't dwell on things.

I certainly don't dwell on things.

The one thing I think about most of all is "What more can we do to help these people?" That's about all.

Chapter 7: *"Listen & Have Compassion"*

What inspires you when you get up each day?

I've got a purpose in life again. And for all those years I had nothing. I'd lost everything, and I didn't have a thing to look forward to. Now I've got a real purpose. People ring me up and ask me to help them.

One of the nicest things was a lady only a few months ago. I'd been helping her son through a depression and he's kind of coming good now. She wrote a letter the other day, and in part of it, she said, "Thank you for giving me back my son." She thought she'd completely lost him.

The sad thing is, even parents don't understand depression. They think that their sons or daughters are lazy or just, you know. But it's not that way at all. If you've ever had depression, all your energy goes, and what energy you've got left, you're keeping that to fight to stay alive, and you don't mean to be angry or lazy.

Some people can't even get out of bed for days and days and days. Some people think depression is when they have a break-up from their girlfriend or boyfriend or something like that, they are just mood things. Then you've got your marriage break-ups or loss of jobs, and that's part of life. When you get into that clinical sort of depression, that's the monster. And, boy, it's time to take action.

When was the point that you said "I'm not going to accept this. I want to do something?"

That's what action means to me. I think the best assets you've got in life are your family.

My situation is a bit strange because my family walked away, except my wife and my mother. I think they might have thought it was contagious or something, because mental illness does scare people.

People are frightened of it. People that I've known for years and years on the farm, they just avoid me, because they'd think "That guy's nuts now".

I was fighting for my life, you know. It's very hurtful when people walk on the other side of the street so they don't have to confront you. That's, I suppose, one of the hardest things, when people misjudge you.

That's compassion. How are we to know what's going on in someone else's life?

You are the only one who knows what's going on in your own head anyway.

I'm not a great believer in drugs and things like that. I think talking to people; sitting there holding hands with someone, you know, or something like that—yeah, that does work. Sitting there talking to your dog, like I used to do. Horses are absolutely incredible with understanding human moods. You can talk to a horse; I don't care what anyone says.

I agree. There are many stories where animals have saved people's lives. They have sensitivity and a dog loves you regardless of what's going on.

Yes, a simple thing like that. Just having another living thing around to talk to, to pat, to let 'em lick your face or just relate to. You can sit there with a dog, and you can cry, and you can cuddle it, and you can do what you like and they're not going to laugh at you. That's the beautiful thing about animals; they just have it all over humans, I reckon.

How can people learn more about Aussie Helpers?

We get a lot of visits on our website. It's currently being updated with all the floods and fires. That's why we're so busy at the moment. It's incredible. I've just come back from around the Echuca area. I've got a list of people to go and see, to talk to. The people who won't go and see a doctor, but they'll talk to me. To me that means respect to me. I'm an ordinary person, just a person.

Chapter 7: *"Listen & Have Compassion"*

A person who is understanding.

They can relate to me because I know a bit about the land and what they are doing and I know what their problems are. I think a lot of these people are frightened to go and see a doctor because they're going to laugh at them. Honestly, there are still a lot of doctors that don't understand depression. I'm not kidding.

People in the bush, they trust me now, and trust other people at Aussie Helpers, because most of us have been down that road, or down some deep well, and swum back up to the top again. We can relate to them. Everything we do is confidential; we're not going to talk about them or anything.

How is it best to contact Aussie Helpers?

If they need help with talking to someone, you ring 1-300-665-232.
Somebody will talk to you straight away.
We'll just listen to your stories, and if you need somebody to go out and see you, we do.
I've driven ten to twelve hours to go out and see people. But we do see them.
The website is **http://www.aussiehelpers.org.au**

Or you can email: admin@aussiehelpers.org.au

At this stage Aussie helpers are in six states, Qld, NSW, Vic, South Australia, Tasmania and also Western Australia.

We can also supply a DVD of Brian Egan on Australian Story and the audio of Murray Hardin's "Rain from Nowhere".

What can people do to help Aussie Helpers if they want to?

To help Aussie Helpers- we don't get government funding or anything- money is what keeps us rolling along. We use a lot of it because the distances and places we go to.
This thing we're doing down the border and into Victoria, this is going to cost a bit, sixty-seventy thousand dollars or something. We'll be carting stock fodder down from Queensland.

We've been lucky. Because of the people we've helped in Southern Queensland over the years, when we asked them to help the people down there with the drought and the fire, they've given us over a quarter of a million dollars worth of stock feed.

That's just the way the wheel turns. That's the bush I suppose.
You help people when they need help, and when you need help, they help you.

Is there anything that we haven't covered that you want to add to help people overcome day-to-day challenges in their life, or to find a purpose and direction?

I think the best advice for people, if they think they've got depression, or if they're showing any signs, is to pick up the phone.

If you're lacking concentration or just the inability to make decisions and things like that, you've got to talk to somebody.

Talk to your wife, or your mate, or your doctor, or just talk to someone.

I mean that, that's the most important thing, and that's what people don't do.

They think…they're ashamed of it.

I was a prime example. I was probably more content to get rid of myself than to go and seek help.

Another one of the good things that helps to use a bit of energy up is a bit of exercise, too.

A simple bit of walking. While you're walking you are going to come across someone; you're going to say "Good day" to them. Walking and talking, I think it's the most important thing on this earth—not to isolate yourself, not to be ashamed of what you think is happening to you. It's so common, it's just a joke now; a terrible joke.

Chapter 7: *"Listen & Have Compassion"*

The Dalai Lama says he wants more friends, because he loves smiles. By making more friends, that's how you get more smiles, but, in particular, a genuine smile.

Oh! That's right.

I think people are better off with a simple life than what's happened in the last few years, with all the material stuff. I think that that's what's isolated a lot of people. Just by not talking; you know, people text message people and send emails, and people forget how to write letters, and post them, and how to pick up a normal telephone and just talk to people, or talk over the back fence, and stuff like that. Those things are gone. It's all cyber sort of stuff.

With all of the upheavals in the world, it actually does bring people together to talk, and work together. It's such a shocking way for that to happen, but it does actually make people talk.

Yeah, and that's so important.

We do a bit of stuff with homeless kids. I was talking to these kids in the street—and I gave this little girl, just 14 years old that day, a hug, and asked why she had left home. The usual answer is they had to leave because they'd been physically or sexually abused by their parents, because of drugs and stuff.

Anyway this kid, just turned fourteen, I gave her a big hug and she said, "Geez, Mr. Egan, that's the first time somebody's given me a hug like that and I didn't have to do anything for it."

Ah, that sort of brings you back to reality. I think we're just losing that but people need to be hugged, and have their hands held, and so forth.

It's coming back to the basics of being human, talking to each other.

Yeah, we'll win in the end.

I think we are winning Brian. I think there are more people who are genuine, honest and caring.

Yeah. Victoria—the bush fires down there—that certainly showed that up. You know, it was horrendous. I'll be back down there this week.

Thank you very much for your time today, Brian.

All right, Trace. Good to talk to you, mate.

ASK WHAT & HOW QUESTIONS

1. Ask What more can I do to help .....?
2. Ask How can I help?
   What skills or knowledge do you have?
3. What are you passionate about?
   Desire alone is strong enough to move mountains.
   When your heart is driven for the best outcome for all involved, start taking the 1st step and you may be amazed at what you can achieve.
4. Take the first step, one step at a time, and follow your passion. Trust yourself.

SIMPLE KINDNESS & COMPASSION MEDITATION DAILY

Sit comfortably, spine straight, feet and legs uncrossed.
Close your eyes, take a DEEP BREATH IN & as you exhale
LET GO and RELAX.
Take another DEEP BREATH IN, focus on your heart.
As you exhale LET GO even further, LET GO of any self judgement,
self criticism, self hatred.
Take another DEEP BREATH IN, focus on your heart.
BREATHE OUT- focus on your heart.

Say the following or similar to yourself:
I care about those in need of assistance.
I send love to my fellow brothers and sisters, 4-legged, 2-legged,
winged and all creatures on the land.
I send love and compassion with all my heart to be with ... that they may ...

Simply be with that uniting connection via Meditation.
Feel the connection with our fellow human beings.
We are not here alone. We are not separate. We can feel their plight.
Our thoughts and hearts are with you.

Slowly open your eyes and be thankful for all you do have.
Be kind and compassionate to yourself too.

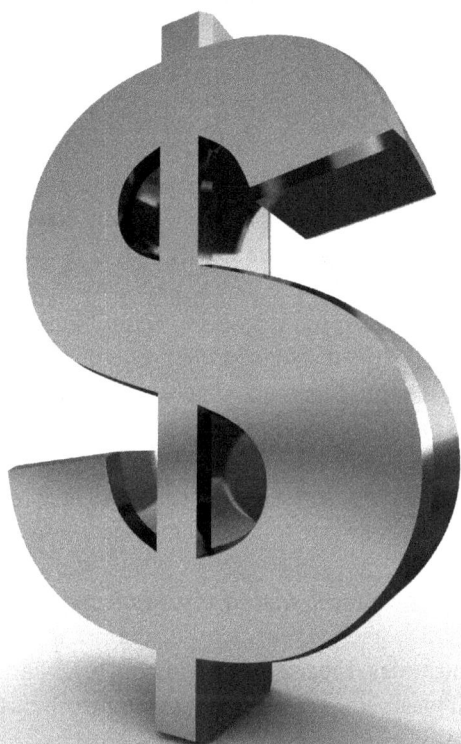

Chapter 8:
"Millionnaire Mindset"

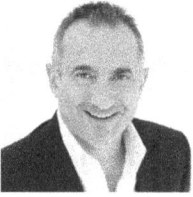

Chapter 8:

"Millionnaire Mindset"

Pat Mesiti

Pat, can you tell us about your background, where you started and where you are now?

I was born into a working class Italian family in Bankstown, Sydney. One of my teachers in high school told me that I would never amount to anything and most likely end up in jail or dead.

I had a very violent home life. Growing up in this kind of environment robs you of security and a sense of self-respect. Not only that, it made me very angry, at my parents, the world and myself.

By the time I was in my teens the violence and drinking at home had worsened. This kind of upbringing meant I had a lot of negative attitudes. I reacted by becoming angry and violent. Some people said it was a stage I was going through, others just pointed and blamed my family.

I had every reason to accept this as "my lot in life". But I saw what was going on around me and had a pretty good idea of where it was going to take me. That caused me to make the decision to "break out". I broke out because I didn't want to be a victim of my own circumstances.

Since I made this decision I have turned my life around completely from growing up in a violent alcoholic family to have my own loving and nurturing environment.

My passion is to help people get what they want out of life. For this to happen, you first have to decide what you actually want. To get the most out of life we have to take charge. I now spend my life helping people of all ages and professions make changes to their own lives. As a motivational speaker I inspire business groups and successful leaders with my incredible life story and positive attitude to live a life of greatness!

Chapter 8: *"Millionnaire Mindset"*

Pat, congratulations on the launch of your latest book "The $1 Million Reason to Change Your Mind." Tell me more about the work you do now and the Millionaire Mindset?

This book is all about helping you to shift your thinking from a poverty mindset to a millionaire mindset. It isn't just about financial prosperity—it's also about mental and emotional wealth; it's about abundance and success in every area of your life. Prosperity definitely includes financial wealth, but it should never be limited to this. Prosperity is something that affects your whole life.

My belief is that every one of us is meant to enjoy a prosperous life. We were never meant only to exist—we are born to live! Our lives are meant to advance.

How many times in your life have you dreamed about what it would be like to be wealthy? Many people spend their whole lives wishing they had more money but never doing anything about it (buying a weekly Lotto ticket doesn't count!) The truth is you can live a more prosperous life if you are prepared to make some changes in your life.

The first place that change needs to happen is in your mind. Before you can become a millionaire, you need to develop the mindset of a millionaire.

If you want to prosper, then there's only one person that matters—you! **You have to decide that you are going to be a wealthy person**. Once you've decided to be a prosperous person and committed yourself to prosperity, you need to learn to focus on that goal, to give attention to the pursuit of prosperity. Your life will follow the direction of your focus.

Whatever you focus on is what will manifest in your life. It's not enough simply to desire to be prosperous. Many people desire things—to be happy, to have a great marriage, to make money—but most stop at desire. Unfortunately, desire alone doesn't get results.

First, you have to think differently about yourself. You need to start seeing yourself as a person who can prosper. You may need to change some ingrained thinking patterns, or perhaps you'll need to overcome negative mindsets that have developed as a result of things that have happened to you in the past.

You might also need to change how you think about wealth and money.

Second, you have to change your thinking about the future. **The future is not predetermined. Rather, we create our futures by the decisions and choices we make today.** What we need is a dream, a clear vision of the future we want to create.

> **Finally, you might need to change the way you think about other people. Instead of seeing others as being in competition with us, or as obstacles we need to negotiate on our way to personal success, we need to see other people as part of the key to our own success.**

My success and prosperity are largely dependent on my associations with and connections to other people.

Can you talk about self esteem?

A critical factor in developing a millionaire mindset is to develop a healthy view of yourself.

How do you see yourself?

Do you see yourself as a person who deserves to prosper, a person who has the potential and the ability to become prosperous?

Or do feel 'unworthy' of prosperity?

Perhaps you think that prosperity is beyond you, that you 'don't have what it takes'. Sterling W. Still said this: **"Wealth is not only what you have but it is also what you are"**. The reason many people don't prosper is not because of their lack of ability or their circumstances but rather because of who they are, or more precisely, who they think or feel they are and how they see themselves. The level of prosperity in your life will be determined to a large extent by who you are as a person.

Chapter 8:   *"Millionnaire Mindset"*

To be prosperous, you need a clear picture of the person you believe you can be. **You will naturally gravitate towards the dominant image of yourself in your mind**. If thoughts of anxiety are your dominant mindset, then you'll gravitate towards anxiety. It's like trying to hit a dartboard with a dart when you're facing another direction. To hit a target you must be facing the direction of the target and focusing on the target.

The biggest hindrance to prosperity is not a lack of money. It's a wrong mindset. Change how you see yourself and others. Your life will not be able to advance until your mind is set to advance.

Ask yourself these questions:
"Do I really value myself?"
"What value do you place on your mind and your knowledge?"
"Do you baulk at the cost of attending a seminar that might help you improve your mind?"

If you truly value yourself, you won't think twice about spending money on self-improvement because your mindset will be not "that's a luxury I can't justify," but rather, "I am worth it!"

To develop a millionaire mindset you need to see yourself in a new light. If you've always thought of yourself as a pauper, start seeing yourself as a prince. If you don't value yourself as much as your should, then start to speak differently about yourself and act differently towards yourself. Go and buy yourself a nice tie or a new dress. Tell yourself that you deserve it, that you are worth it.

"But," I hear you ask, "Isn't it really more important to value other people? Shouldn't my motivation to be wealthy be so that I can help others?" My answer is "yes", but it is not possible to value other people any more than you value yourself.

One of the great principles of the Christian faith is the requirement to "love your neighbour as yourself". This implies that you can only love your neighbour if you first love yourself. A millionaire mindset places a high value on self and then turns that outward by placing equally high value on other people.

What was the turning point in your life?

At one time in my life, I suffered from depression for over eighteen months.

Then one day I had what could almost be described as an awakening where I started to think, "I don't want to be depressed anymore".

As a result of this change of mindset, I managed to throw off my depression.

Depression is a state of mind, not an emotional state. Depression results from a thought pattern that is all about hopelessness and gloom. To get rid of depression you need to change the way you think.

What was the thought process that turned that around?

Change begins in the mind. The mind is like a filter through which we interpret the world and our own experiences and form our beliefs, attitudes and understanding of the nature of 'reality'.

No two people see a single situation the same way. The classic illustration of this is the difference between the person who sees the glass as half empty and the one who sees the same glass as half full—same glass, different perspectives. Why the difference? Because the minds of the two observers are filtering the information they are receiving about the glass of water differently. We would label the first person as a pessimist and the second as an optimist.

Did you grow up in a home where all you ever heard from your parents were expressions like

"We're not made of money" or
"Money doesn't grow on trees, you know"?

Chapter 8: *"Millionnaire Mindset"*

Or perhaps your view of money is even more severe. Maybe you grew up hearing things like

"Money is the root of all evil"or

"Money ruined my marriage".

If your mindset is that money is always incredibly hard to come by, or that money is somehow inherently evil, then before you can truly prosper you will need to change your philosophy about money. Our outward behaviour will always conform to our internal mindset. That means if we want to change how we act, we first have to change how we think.

In order to bring about change in your external world, you have to work on your mind, your attitudes, the way you think about and construct your life.

In your day-to-day life are you playing offence or defence?

Are you waiting for your lucky break or are you busy creating your future?

Are you focused on end results or on the process?

Are you blaming your past or confronting it?

You cannot change what you won't confront.

Be aware of why you think the way you think. Thought patterns can be deep rooted and you have to be aware of them and where they came from. There are some thought patterns and focuses in our lives that we need to uproot if we are ever to become prosperous.

As the saying goes, "if you want to fly with the eagles, don't hang out with the turkeys".

What is the first step in making a mindset shift?

It starts with awareness. You need to become aware of how you think and why you think the way you think.

Once you've developed this awareness about your thinking you are in a position to change how you think. If you change your thinking, it will change how you feel; if you change your feelings, it will change how you act; if you change your actions, it will change your level of prosperity. It's a five-stage process:

Awareness > Think > Feel > Act > Live

Words we speak can also have a significant influence on our mindsets. We need to pay close attention to the things we say about and the words we allow to dominate important areas of our lives such as our relationships, our financial world and our physical wellbeing. Words have the power to create or destroy us.

When we speak positively about our lives, we reinforce positive mindsets and therefore generate positive feelings, which in turn lead to positive actions that have a positive impact on our lives.

You can start building a millionaire mindset today simply by starting to speak positively about yourself and your world. If negative words have brought you down or held you back in the past, then you can change that today by neutralising the power of those words.

If someone has told you you're no good, start telling yourself what a great person you are. If you've been told it's impossible or you'll never make it, start telling yourself that you are going to make it, that it can be done and you are going to do it. If you've been told that you're just average, start telling yourself that you are outstanding, way above average. If there are things in your world that you want to see change, start talking about those things as though they are changing.

There is a story of two shoe salesmen who go to Africa. One of them quickly writes back to his employer: "Please send me a ticket home. I have no hope of selling shoes here because nobody here wears shoes." The other salesman also writes home: "Please send me a thousand pairs of shoes as soon as you can. There is a great opportunity for us because nobody here wears shoes!" Same experience, different responses. Why? Because they think differently. They have different mindsets.

Make up your mind today to change your mind. Start thinking bigger. Expand your capacity. Begin seeing the world around you as being full of opportunity rather than impossibility. That's a millionaire mindset.

Chapter 8:   *"Millionnaire Mindset"*

Expect things to go well, expect yourself to prosper, expect to be wealthy, expect to be on time, expect to lose weight, expect to be healthy, expect to develop great friendships.

If you focus your attention on making excuses, then your excuses will flourish; if you focus on creating wealth, then that will expand. If you spend your mental energy on constantly worrying, excusing and justifying, it will be difficult, if not impossible, to create abundance in your life.

Are you in the habit of making excuses? If you are stop it! **You were designed for advancement, you were engineered for prosperity and you have been endowed with seeds of greatness.**

What does it mean to have a millionaire mindset on a daily basis?

- Having a millionaire mindset means you play to win as opposed to simply playing not to lose.
- A person with a millionaire mindset is a person who is constantly asking questions and finding answers. Unlike the person with a poverty mindset, they don't assume that they already know it all. They are inquisitive, not constantly opinionated. Rather than being an armchair expert, a prosperity thinker is always learning something new.
- The millionaire mindset is able to ignore criticism. I don't listen to my critics; I listen to my mentors and leaders, the people I have given permission to speak into my life.
- A person with a millionaire mindset goes beyond desire to commitment. It's not enough just to want to be prosperous—you have to be passionately committed to becoming prosperous.
- People with a millionaire mindset have a different understanding of their personal worth. They develop their self worth before they develop their net worth.
- To have a millionaire mindset is to recognise the need for mentors, people you can look up to and seek guidance and inspiration from. These are people who have been successful and achieved things that you are still aiming to achieve.
- Millionaire mindset people use what is in their hand to do what's in their heart. People with a poverty mindset are not driven by what's in their heart and as a result their hands are tied. People like Sir Bob Geldof and U2 front man Bono are passionate about causes such as the elimination of poverty in the world. They have used their celebrity as rock stars to try to influence world leaders to bring about change, as was evidenced by the recent 'Live 8' global rock concert.

Start by asking yourself:
What's in your heart? What's your dream? What's your passion?
Now ask yourself this:
"What do I have in my hand today that I can utilise to start moving in the direction of what's in my heart?"

- Another important characteristic of the millionaire mindset is the quality of courage.
- Think of success, not failure. In taking risks, understand what the probable outcomes will be. Then do whatever you can to improve the chance of getting the outcome you desire.
- Believing in yourself and being prepared to work hard are two ways of reducing fear and anxiety and bolstering your courage.
- To build your belief in yourself, prepare and plan for success, focus on the key issues and be well organised.
- Playing competitive sports is a good way to develop the mental toughness needed to handle fear. Develop an "athlete's heart." It's all about developing "physical and mental tenacity and courage."
- Strong religious faith is an important factor for almost 40 percent of the millionaires surveyed. Those who have some kind of strong faith exhibit a higher propensity to take financial risks.

What is the most important advice anyone has given you?

One of the greatest lessons I have ever learnt is that the key to wealth and prosperity and making money is to solve problems and troubles. Anyone who has ever created wealth has been in the problem-solving business. People like Bill Gates or Henry Ford to name just a couple— people like this make money because they solve problems.

Money has no mystical or mysterious powers to turn people either into corrupt capitalists or virtuous paupers. It is what is in the heart of a person that renders that person's money either good or bad. In the drug addict's hand it will be used to support bad habits, but in the prosperous person's hand it will be spread about and invested wisely.

What else has been important for you going forward?

You might have a dream and hit every goal you set for yourself, but a dream in and of itself is not enough. Unless you are able to change your mindset to think how wealthy people think—to think with a millionaire mindset—you won't achieve sustainable prosperity.

Chapter 8: *"Millionnaire Mindset"*

How can people learn more from you?

Visit Pat Mesiti's Motivational Minute at **http://www.mesiti.com**

What are you passionate about in your life?

I am passionate about being a compassionate capitalist! In other words, I have prosperity for a purpose. My money, your money, our money can accomplish great things. With money, we can make the world a better place.

> What are you concerned about?
> What moves you? What flicks your switch?
> What makes you angry? What makes you exuberant? What makes you feel a sense of drive? What makes you burn with fervour?

This is not about feelings; this is a disposition we need to have. We need to develop a passionate disposition about creating wealth for ourselves and for others.

Above all, you have to keep believing—no matter what. You have to believe that dreams come true.

Are there any final thoughts you would like to offer to help others overcome stress in their life?

Adversity causes some people to break, but others to break records.

Anyone who wants to prosper and increase, to flourish and advance, must consider what they have now and work on that, and not complain about what they have lost, what could have been, might have been or should have been. Such complaining is pointless and energy draining and a prosperity thief.

Welcome to the human race! Everybody has baggage. Everyone has made mistakes. Everyone has been hurt or treated badly at one time or another. If you've messed up or been messed up at any time in your life then you are the perfect candidate for success. You've got to get over your past.

Many people get stuck in the past because they are continually looking in the rear vision mirror of their life. You cannot go forward while ever you are constantly looking backwards.

What do you really want in life? I want to prosper. I want to create wealth. I want to help other people become wealthy. I want to help people who are disadvantaged to go to another level, and to do that I need money.

If your life were a blank canvas in front of you what would you want to put on it?
What's your family like?
What are your kids like?
What's your career like?
What's your world like?
How would you think?
How would you feel?
How would you speak?
How would you live?

Once you've figured out exactly what you want, the next challenge is to stay focused on it.

Focus can be incredibly powerful. It can help us to overcome seemingly insurmountable obstacles and bring about change in the face of what might seem like overwhelming adversity.

As I've said, what you focus on will progress and what you neglect will regress. Many people get sick because they neglect their bodies—smoking, poor eating habits, lack of exercise, not enough sleep.

A change of focus can turn around years of neglect. If someone in poor physical condition decides they want to be healthy and then gets focused on becoming healthy, then change will happen. As they give up smoking, start eating well, begin exercising regularly and generally begin to live a wholesome lifestyle, their physical condition begins to improve. Why? Because you get what you focus on.

Chapter 8: *"Millionnaire Mindset"*

Developing a millionaire mindset requires a focused mind. Spend some time each day forcing yourself to focus your mind on the things that matter in your world.

Growth is a process, not an event. Growth has nothing to do with your age; it is all about your desire for success.

If the desire for something greater doesn't drive you to change, then a crisis generally will.

The exciting truth in all this is that the starting point of the quest for a millionaire mindset is wherever you are right now. No matter who you are, or what you know or don't know about money and wealth, or what your current circumstances are, or what has happened to you in the past, if you simply make a firm decision today to do something to change your world, then you are at the starting point of seeing increase and prosperity in your life.

What is in your heart of hearts?
What is the thing that you long to do in your wildest dreams?
How big can you make this thing called your life?

When it comes to developing a millionaire mindset, you have to love your dream and love what you are doing to make your dream a reality. If you don't love what you are doing, then do something else! Vision is always emotional. Everyone has a different vision because everyone gets excited by different things.

Focus on your gift. Don't function and expect prosperity to come from outside of your gift. Work on your strengths. Vision has to involve passion and motivation.

Start today.

ASK WHAT & HOW QUESTIONS

Ask yourself these questions today:

1. How can I change my behaviour so I fly with the Eagles?
2. What gift do I have? Everyone is good at something.
   What are you great at doing?
3. What are you passionate about?
   What moves you?
   What inspires you?

When you are clear about what you want, then FOCUS and you shall surely succeed.

Step by Step.

SOW THE SEEDS AT NIGHT AS YOU GO TO BED
THE MIRACLE QUESTION

How do I go about changing the way I think? One strategy you can adopt is a therapeutic technique called the 'miracle question'. It goes like this:

Imagine that when you go to bed tonight and while you are asleep a miracle happens. The effect of this miracle is that the problems that brought you here are resolved, but you don't know this because you are still asleep.

When you awake tomorrow morning, what will be the first thing you notice that will tell you that this problem is resolved?

The idea of this technique is to help you begin thinking differently about your life and begin to imagine what your world could be like.

The simple solution is to start thinking and acting as though things have changed today.

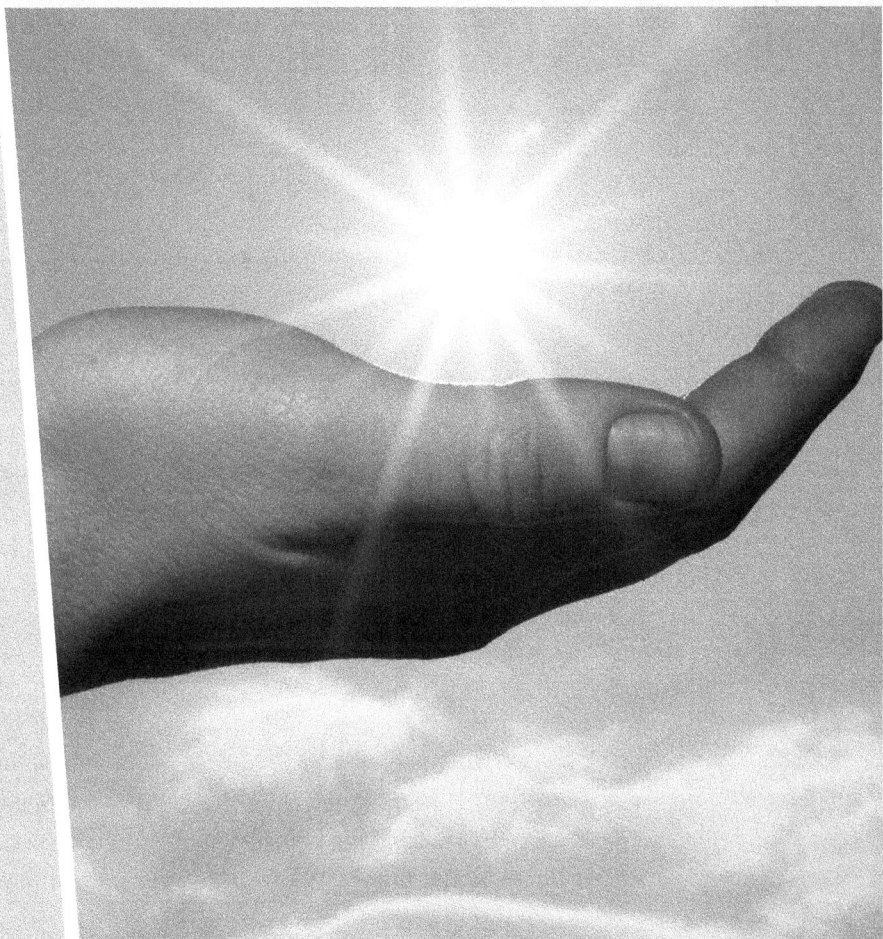

Chapter 9:

Learning to Accept Help
from Others

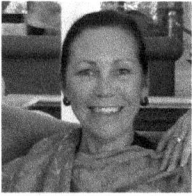

Chapter 9:

Learning to Accept Help from Others
Mukti Lartigau

Mukti, can you tell us about your background and how you have overcome stress naturally?

I've been a natural therapist for about thirty years. I've been a yoga instructor for about the same time. I became very interested in meditation, and probably I've been teaching for about twenty years.

I became interested when I realised how stressed most people are in their daily lives. I mean, just getting in the car in the morning and driving through traffic is stressful and we take all that for granted. I decided that we need to be meditating on a day-to-day basis. I was teaching my yoga classes twice a week and doing long one-hour meditations during that time.

People were staggering through the door and saying things like "I've only just made it through the week to get back to this – let's meditate now." I did guided visualizations with times of complete silence, but mainly people anchored themselves to my voice, because the mind wanders.

Then when my painful situation started about eleven months ago, I got into meditation with a real vengeance because it took me into places that I needed to go because of the pain that I was going through in my own body.

The first thing that was happening was that they were realising how powerful the mind is and that it takes you to where it wants you to go, not particularly where you want to go.

Chapter 9: *Learning to Accept Help from Others*

What was it that happened eleven months ago?

I got bulging discs right at the top of my spine. I always had a problem with what they refer to the Hangman's Break which was at the top of my neck from a childhood incident.

Now I have massive spine degeneration from behind my breasts up, the whole cervical spine. There is no space between any of the discs. Further down along my back there are more bulging discs. I would lie down then try to get up again but my knees had gone, I couldn't move. It was as if everything had hit me at once. I think it was a bit of osteoarthritis. Had I not done the yoga that I'd been doing for thirty years, I would not have had the muscle in the top of my neck and across my shoulders to support that crumbling spine. And now, of course, I don't have those muscles because I haven't been able to do anything for about eleven months.

Was it something in particular that triggered the physical pain?

I think age, probably. I lifted something very heavy that I shouldn't have lifted, and I think that popped the bulging discs out further. That was excruciating pain. Once again, I'm dealing with it myself, the way I dealt with it in the very beginning when I was diagnosed with this Hangman's Break. I've been to a couple of different practitioners, and then thought about what they told me and then I have gone my own way mineralizing the body and rebuilding all of the bones and the spine. It's what I think I can do. Well, what I know I can do. I am taking lots of extra minerals, a lot of vegetable juices.

Did you educate yourself on what you needed to do?

Yes, I've been educated for a long time and telling other people, but of course, when it comes to you, turning that caring onto yourself, turning the focus into yourself, I found it to be one of the most difficult things. It is probably why my bones began to degenerate, it was my need to do exactly that - turn the focus in on myself. It certainly stopped me in my tracks, I worked very hard and very long hours, with many people, and I guess the universe just hits you on the head if you are not paying attention to yourself. So this really got my attention. Pain does that.

What was the journey you went through emotionally, that the pain led you through?

Ah, frustration, a kind of non-belief that it was actually happening to me. Certainly my clients were all blown away. The fact that this strong woman who usually did everything for everybody else, who worked and taught yoga, had just been felled. It doesn't make sense. And, of course, I wondered about my own ability to be able to advise other people, given what was actually happening to me. I had to get myself over that, as well.

Did it affect your self-esteem?

Well… yes and no, because very quickly I got to the point of realising that this was very necessary, and it was, in fact, a gift. And a lot of my clients, in fact, most of them realised that as well. So, here I had it… a hole in one.

A gift in what way?

It is an absolute knowing that everything we draw in we are the directors on the stage, the stage of my life, and we're pulling all these situations in, in order to learn so we never ever have to go through this stuff again.

> **I had to learn to listen to my body, which, at that point in time, I don't think I was doing. There is nothing like pain to focus you.**

You can actually go inside pain. I can imagine that for some people it would be quite addictive, because it cocoons you. I'm sure a lot of women in childbirth will agree, you can go into this place and it's like you get behind the pain, and you operate from there.

I can understand why people would go into deep depression with something like this. Fortunately I've pinpointed why I haven't. It's because I'm fascinated by it. It is as if I can take one step backwards from myself, and I actually observe what's going on with me. I'm sure that other people can do it too, and I'm also sure that a lot of people can't, because pain is so self-involving.

Chapter 9: *Learning to Accept Help from Others*

I am more fascinated with the pain than depressed with it.

Can you tell me how you've learnt to listen to your body more?

I think that has come as a direct result of the pain. That's why I know that it was very necessary, because otherwise I think I would have kept going as I was going. The pain really gives me the horrors, sometimes. It frustrates me and a couple of times I've tossed the cushion across the room, but that's about as far as I've gone. I was so active, and now I'm not. And I will be again. I will. I will. It doesn't feel permanent, this thing.

It feels like an incredible lesson handed to me on a golden platter.

I was pretty well connected to myself, but obviously not connected enough. I think the only thing for this little being, was pain, to get my attention and focus my attention completely.

To come back to yourself?

Yes. To come back to myself and listen. Just lie on the bed and gaze out the window and be very connected with every little thing that was going on. From heartbeat to... I've being in meditative situations where I can feel my blood moving around my body.

You have become more aware... you've learned to listen more to your body... to where the pain is?

Well, firstly, I realised that I've got to be absolutely present in the moment, and yes, watch the pain. If there's a pain in my body I'll focus there and really feel it and try to identify it, and give it a personality. The last three weeks now just before I wake up a whole lot of information drops in, right on waking... sometimes my eyes are actually open and my body will go...B12, you need more B12, and things like that so... I'm really starting to jot things down so I don't forget. I also have the knowledge that it's all about me. It's never about the other. Just me. I'm doing massive backyard clearing at the moment. It ripples out on everyone else, because there's no separation between any of us.

What have you found works best to motivate you and keep you focused each day to overcome the stress caused by the pain?

Having something to do. I found that I'm scheduling myself. I get up in the morning and have a shower and get dressed and… even dressing myself is hard.

All these tiny little steps that before I took for granted, but I don't take for granted anymore.

Then I go out and do some shopping, and I park away from the shops so that I can walk. I am absolutely exhausted when I get home. I do try to stay out for about three hours before I go home and get on the bed. Getting myself up and having a bit of routine, and having my meditations every morning and keeping things the same, it all helps.

I make sure that I'm taking minerals and natural foods, and I like it. I have breakfast now instead of racing out. I am now forced to be looking at me and what is good for me. It's obvious to me now what is actually going on.

What would you say was the turning point in coming to an understanding?

A hell of a lot happened in that twelve months. I was working, and then I did a course, teaching English. I actually went to Vietnam with this injury. For some reason I thought I would get better when I got over there, and I'll have lots to do and, of course it got worse. I ended up having to buy a walking stick, and my knees were pretty bad at that point. My knees are actually OK now.

Since I got back from Vietnam, I did have to be helped off the aircraft in a wheelchair because I'd been sitting for so long, life has looked up since then. Then I went to Bundaburg to a friend's place, we ran a cancer clinic together near Byron Bay years ago. I knew I had to be with them, that I would be fed properly and looked after to go through my process to reassemble myself and handle what was coming up emotionally.

Chapter 9: *Learning to Accept Help from Others*

I did that for a length of time. Then my dad got sick and I decided to come back down to the Gold Coast.

I think there was a turning point there, because I learned how to live day by day with this pain, and also learned how to feed myself. Not that the feeding of myself was greatly different to what I had always done, but I upped the ante with vegetable juice daily, and lots more minerals, making sure that everything that went into my mouth was organic, where possible, and highly mineralized.

You said another turning point was when you came back down to the Gold Coast?

Yes, I'm having little turning points all the time. Little turning points are happening probably every week. As I understand things. Maybe I can't sit for too long, which tells me I am not meant to. I'm meant to be moving. I think it's hotting up on the planet. And I think I have always had the knowing that I am here for something quite specific, and that my learning is quite focused and for a reason. I think that reason is going to be revealed in the next few years. I need to be strong for that because I think there are people on the planet who will need guidance from people who are not run by their ego minds. People who are coming from their hearts with the highest possibility and greatest good.

What has been your biggest lesson from this dis-ease in your body?

Accepting help from other people. I was always the one who helped others. Learning to say no was a big thing and accepting help from people.

Sometimes I would almost be teary saying no to people. I realised that physically I could not do it. That was huge for me. Huge.

It's one thing to say "Yes I accept help from others", but do we really?

Well obviously I didn't. The state I am in at the moment, physically, I decided, is the only state I could possibly be in to learn what I needed to learn. I am very grateful for it, really. I say that in the morning now. When I am in the greatest pain I say "I am so grateful for this".

What is the most important advice that someone has ever given to you?

Just going inside, I think. I was blessed having the grandmother that I had. She was a Buddhist. Her own brand of Buddhism. She was, I would say, my first mentor. She said things like "You are the centre of the universe." You might think that's what all grandmothers say to their grandchildren, but she meant "Everything there is to know is inside of you."

All you have to do is be still, and silent and the information will be given to you.

There is nothing that you can learn. The older I get the more I realise how we run interference on ourselves, we block ourselves from the knowledge that we have innately in our heart, in the bones and cells of our body. We get caught up in this day to day illusion that we call our lives.

What inspires you each day to keep going?

I see things here, on the Gold Coast. I mean visually, people laugh at me when I talk about the light on the Gold Coast. When I look back towards the Hinterland, and when I look out my bedroom window, the light is beautiful. It's quite incredible.

Trees. I have a huge connection with trees.
Books. I'm inspired all the time by books, by the people who write books and can say things in a way that's so succinct, and to the point and focused. I'm very inspired by people who can get a message out in just a few words. You know, I think people are so clever. It's not

clever… they are coming from their heart and speaking
the truth. That's why it's inspirational.

Thank you for speaking from your heart Mukti and sharing your
journey and lessons.

AWARENESS / MINDFULNESS DAILY ACTIVITIES

1. What are you grateful for in your life? Write it down.
2. Can you turn "your pain" into a gift? How can you shift
   your perception to see your pain as a gift? What lesson is
   the gift for you to know? Write it down.
3. You have the answers within you. Trust your intuition.
   Trust your knowing. Be still so you can hear the answers
   to your questions. Be aware of your monkey thoughts,
   your intuition, your inner knowing. You know the
   difference. Trust yourself. We all know when we know.
   It's a knowing feeling.

   Everyone can experience a knowing feeling that
   comes from within. Within our heart and soul.

"The trick is in what one emphasizes. We either make ourselves miserable, or we make ourselves happy. The amount of work is the same."
Carlos Castaneda

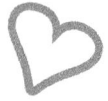

HEALING MEDITATION

Choose to take care of your body. Listen to your body. How can you nourish and nurture your body? How can you help to heal your body? Ask – and ye shall receive, in the stillness of Mind.

Sit comfortably, spine straight, feet and legs uncrossed.
Close your eyes, take a DEEP BREATH IN.
As you exhale LET GO of the day, LET GO of all thoughts, LET GO of all emotions.
Take another DEEP BREATH IN, focus only on your breathing.
As you exhale LET GO even further, LET GO and RELAX, LET GO of everything.
Take another DEEP BREATH IN, focus only on the breath.
Exhale, focus only on the breath.
As you continue to BREATHE DEEPLY IN & OUT, focus your awareness on the part of your body that is "hurting".
ENERGY follows AWARENESS. Keep your Awareness on the "pain" in your body and HEALING ENERGY will flow to that part of your body.

In the stillness of Mind, say repeatedly to yourself this Healing Chant:

I heal my body, I heal my mind
With love that nurtures and love that's kind
The power that made me is mine to use
To heal me or hurt me, whichever I choose.

The human body is truly amazing – we can heal ourselves.

Go to <u>www.HowToOvercomeStressNaturally.com/Resources</u>
to listen to the Healing Chant

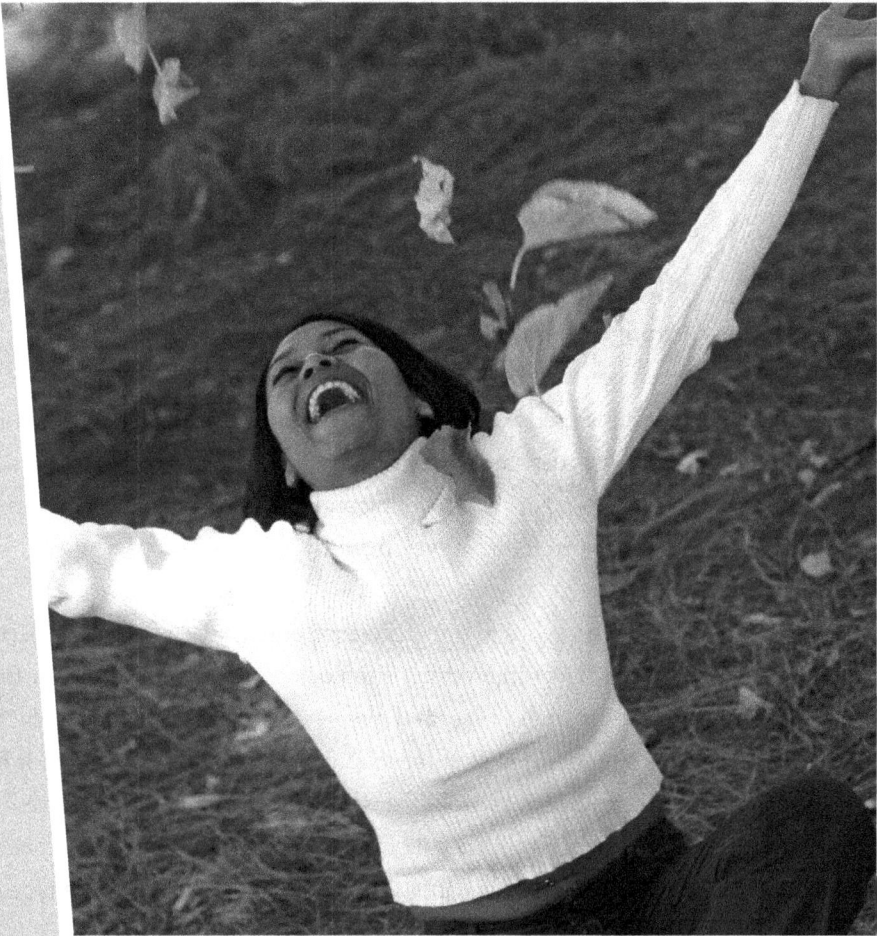

Chapter 10:

*A Spark Inside eventually led
me out of Depression*

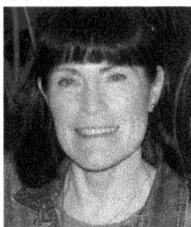

Chapter 10:

A Spark Inside eventually led me out of Depression

Elizabeth Joy

Elizabeth, tell us about your background and your journey through stress and depression.

Like most people I've had ups and downs and challenges in my life. I felt I had become a very positive, happy and healthy person. My life was going well. I was working and following my passion. I was getting into my writing and developing my spiritual and psychic self.

About 10 years ago my biggest experience with stress and depression began when I injured my shoulder and neck and the pain from the injury became worse and worse and nothing I did could heal it. The pain became so intense and went on for so long that it became emotional pain as well. The stress on my body became stress on my mind which eventually became depression. This chronic pain lasted for about 18 months and was very debilitating. It was the type of pain that you would do just about anything to be free of.

Were you able to find a solution to get rid of that physical pain?

No. I tried everything and anything that might help, medical and non medical. But for me nothing could alleviate the pain for long and would aggravate it in some cases. The longer it went on the more stressed I became. No one could tell me why it was getting worse and not better.

Chapter 10: *A Spark Inside eventually led me out of Depression*

At that time what emotions were you going through?

You name them I went through them all. Anger, frustration, disappointment and resentment were just some of the emotions I went through. But fear and sadness became the overriding emotions. Fear that I was never going to get better, fear that I couldn't and wouldn't be able to do the activities I wanted to. Simple things like reading a book and writing were near impossible. Sadness that I couldn't be who I was.

I had to give up work at the time. That was frustrating. I was confused as to why I wasn't healing. I hated the situation I was in so that compounded everything. Because I was normally positive, happy and healthy I think that made it worse because I was used to being able to sort things out in a positive way.

Was the pain overwhelming?

Looking back now the pain did become my main focus. It became overwhelming. I didn't like myself because I wasn't able to overcome the pain or the depression. The more I noticed the pain, the more it seemed to increase. When the pain would subside for a little while, my mind and body would prepare for when it would come back again.

How did that affect your self-esteem?

I couldn't resolve the situation the way I thought I should be able to. I felt powerless. It was a combination of everything that affected my self-esteem.

What was the key for you that started to turn the pain and depression around?

Well it was a very gradual process. I started to focus and listen more to the voice within, a spark inside, a feeling of hope that things could and would get better.

It may sound strange to some when I say I listened to a voice within, a spark inside. There is more to us than just our physical body. I believe we also have a spirit and soul.

Focusing more on the spark of hope I began to slowly accept the situation to make peace with where I was and with what was happening and not happening. I began being easier on myself for getting into the situation and for being depressed.

I slowly stopped fighting the situation and myself.

Embracing my spiritual connection more was important for me. Hope and faith are part of spiritualness. I had to feel more and think less. I had to connect more with my heart and less with my mind.

Was the pain continuing at this point of time?

Most of the time there was pain or discomfort to some degree.
The pain was around my neck and shoulders and every time I used my arm it got aggravated. So I tried not to use my arm. Simple things like using a computer, I couldn't use the mouse for more than a minute or the pain would come back.

What was the thought process that had you do something different than you had done before?

I began slowly to focus less on the pain and little by little more on the moments when the pain would ease. I started to remember those moments more than I was remembering the pain filled moments. I also stopped thinking that the pain and depression was wrong or bad in some way. That helped me to think and feel differently about the situation.

I had to let it be okay to be depressed. I had to let it be okay to take as long as I needed to move through it. It was a very slow process, in fact sometimes I felt I was standing still or even going backwards. That had to be ok as well if I was to keep going at all.

Chapter 10: *A Spark Inside eventually led me out of Depression*

Whatever I was thinking and feeling, I had to be ok with it in some way. That can be challenging if you are somewhere you don't want to be.

Eventually I came to understand that depression is a way the mind tries to cope with a situation and emotions it does not like or want. It's trying somehow to avoid them. It's like it goes into emotional overload. That was true for me because there were so many strong emotions that had built up over time that I was experiencing all together.

You said to yourself that you would heal over time?

Yes, saying that helped but it was feeling and believing that what I was saying was true that gave it power. Giving myself time to do it, step by step not thinking I had to sort it all at once helped. I didn't become depressed overnight so I had to realise it was going to be a gradual process to move through it. I had to let my body and mind heal itself. I had to get out of the way. As my thinking and feelings changed, gradually my physical and emotional pain became less and less.

Did you start looking for different solutions which you hadn't tried before?

The main difference was letting it all be ok no matter what. Not fight the situation. Not putting a time limit on anything. I had to let go of asking myself why me, why now. Why couldn't I overcome the situation?

Nowadays, how do you take control of negative thoughts & emotions on a daily basis?

Ten years ago I didn't have the same awareness and understanding of the mind and emotions I do now. I continue putting in as many positive, inspiring thoughts, sounds and visions as possible. If a thought I don't want to think does appear I don't make it wrong I simply think something I do want to think. I don't make a big deal out of it. My thinking that my pain and depression was wrong or bad in the beginning didn't help matters. The mind works with whatever we put into it.

What have you found works best to keep you motivated and focused each day?

I now practise meditation each day. I keep it simple. It's a wonderful exercise for both mind and body.
That's something that I love doing.

What else has been important for you to keep yourself stress free?

- Having a laugh each day.
  Being able to laugh at myself is a wonderful stress reliever. I can do that more than I used to now. Not taking life or myself too seriously. Well not all the time.
- Having some fun.
- I use meditation as a preventive for stress rather than a cure.
- Being creative in some way I enjoy.
- And having a still moment now and then.

Elizabeth what inspires you each day?

The simplicity of Life. Life is not complicated unless we make it to be. Being creative. Helping others.

You have written a book. Can you tell me about your book?

My book is called *"Reconnect with the Heart and Remember the Soul."* It's a book of spiritual simplicity expressed through poetry, acronyms, affirmations and meditations. It can be used for personal peace and self empowerment.

I believe it is inspired writing on subjects such as Life, Peace, Forgiveness, Birth and Death. I feel my book can help people to become more in harmony with who they are and can further Embrace, Strengthen and Expand their own Spirituality. It is my hope that the reader receives as much inspiration from my book as I did in writing it.

Chapter 10: *A Spark Inside eventually led me out of Depression*

Would you like to share some of your acronyms?

Well HOPE is:

> Hold
> Only
> Positive
> Emotions.

Never give up hope and Hold Only Positive Emotions.

Stress and depression are negative emotions that can be changed to positive emotions, one thought and emotion at a time.

FAITH is:

> Full
> Alignment
> In
> The
> Heart.

When we have Full Alignment In The Heart we can hear our inner voice, the spark, and our own truth.

What else do you find helpful?

- Learn meditation before you need it. The irony is if we learn meditation before we need it, the less we are likely to need it. I know for a fact trying to learn to meditate when you are stressed or depressed can be very challenging to say the least.
- Expressing yourself creatively is a very good way to alleviate stress. It can give the mind something else to focus on other than your problems. Writing my book was my way of expressing my creativity. It was of immense help to me.
- Find something that you are passionate about and interested in and like doing.
- Just have fun with something.
- Keep spiritually connected in any way that feels good to you.
- Waking up in the morning and saying thank you.

Are there any other thoughts you'd like to express to help others with stress and depression which you have not covered already?

- There is always a solution to every challenging situation.
- Be okay with wherever you are, at that moment, even if you're not ok with where you are just yet.
- If we can look at chronic stress as a warning signal letting us know that our thoughts and emotions are taking us in a direction we don't want to go we can do something about it. Continued stress on the mind or body will eventually lead to something unwanted.
- Talking to someone can help. A family member a friend or therapist. Someone you trust who is non-judgemental.
- Talking and listening to your inner self, your spiritual self is the most important thing you can do for yourself. For me having a spiritual belief was very important.
- My mother was a wonderful support and I am grateful to her for that.
- No one can do it for us. We are the only ones that can make ourselves happy, or unhappy.
- Connect with the heart as much as possible by being creative, meditating or having a still moment.
- Do something you love.
- Help someone in need or a charity. There is always someone we can help if we look around. It helps to take our mind of our own problems.
- Life is too short to let worry become stress and stress become depression.
- Remember saying "it's all okay" makes a great mantra.

Do you have a website?

Yes Tracey. It is http://www.elizabethjoy.com.au/
There you can find out a little more about my book and what I now do.

Finally, can you tell me 3 things you are grateful for in your life?

1. The freedom to experience and to express Hope, Faith and Love.
2. The still small voice within.
3. The Spark, of course.

Chapter 10: *A Spark Inside eventually led me out of Depression*

Thank you very much Elizabeth. Thank you for all your advice and your book is very inspirational.

Thank you, Tracey, for allowing me to share my journey. I hope it is of some help to others. I would also like to share a poem I've just written. It's called The Spark Within. So have fun Tracey and enjoy life.

DAILY CREATIVITY

1. What Creative Expression brings you Joy?
- Painting / Drawing
- Playing music / Composing Music
- Writing: a note to a special friend, a play for the theatre one day
- Writing: a story, your daily diary, internal reflection for yourself
- Creative Craftwork
- Hobby that you love, in your creative style
- Playing with the children, grandparents, the family, friends
- Sport: creating a winning team!
- Having fun in any crazy, unique, creative way you want!

2. I would love to hear from you. Write your story of creative joy and fulfilment to: Go To:
    www.HowToOvercomeStressNaturally.com

3. Positively Encourage Your Creativity Daily.
    Creative ideas come to me all the time.
    I am open to receive an abundance of exciting creative ideas.
    I express myself freely and creatively with ease.
    I create the space and time to be creative.

DAILY CONTEMPLATION
TO GROW YOUR SPARK WITHIN

The Spark Within

I walk beside you in the valley of shadows
I hold you close when your world falls apart
I comfort you in your time of sorrow
I speak to you through the voice of your heart

I am the source of the peace that you seek
For I am the spark of hope that you feel
I rejoice with you when you embrace this connection
For I am the spark of faith that can heal

I am the spark that lights the way
When you reach out to me I take your hand
Whatever happens and whatever you do
Remember this always, I understand

For I walk beside you in the valley of shadows
I hold you close when your world falls apart
I comfort you in your time of sorrow
And I listen to you through the voice of your heart.

copyright© Elizabeth Joy 2009

"The deeper sorrow carves into your being the more joy you can contain."
Kahlil Gibran

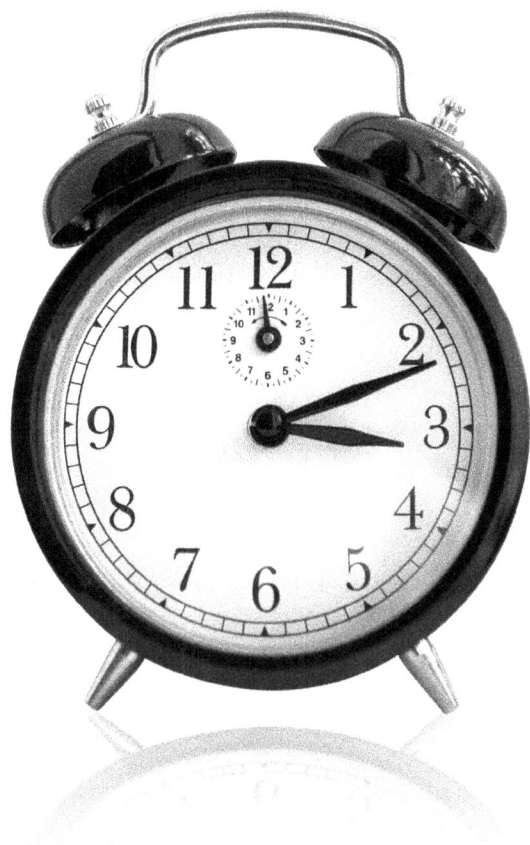

Chapter 11:

"Love & Time the Healer" - A Mum's Journey with her Daughter

Chapter 11:

"Love & Time the Healer" -
A Mum's Journey with her Daughter

"Always bear in mind that your own resolution to succeed is
more important than any other one thing."
Abraham Lincoln

"Wheresoever you go, go with all your heart."
Confucious

Dawn, can you tell us about your daughter's depression and your journey?

In the beginning my daughter Belinda, started to shut herself away a lot from people. It started first with her family, and then it grew to all her friends.

She kept a lot of secrets about how she was feeling.

She could sit and talk to people and look totally at ease and happy, and then go for days where she didn't want to see anyone or go anywhere or do anything. She became a loner. She would just sit for days and not want to see anyone.

She had a partner, who didn't understand what was wrong with her. He would ridicule her, which made her rebel against him. She was trying to explain to him how she felt, but he didn't understand. As a result of that it made her even worse, and in the end, his lack of support and understanding was one of the factors that caused their relationship to break up after six years.

This then sent her spiralling into a deep depression. She tried to cope. She lived on this hope that he would come back to her, but he'd moved on. She had trouble accepting it, and went into a state of suicidal tendencies, and the fact that she wanted to die indicated to me that she was screaming out for help. Belinda could have died because she took a huge overdose.

What actually happened at that time?

At the last minute she told me that she saw my picture on the dressing table, and that made her decide no.

I think she was in such terrible confusion and hurt.

She described the feeling as constant pain, a pain that someone might feel if someone they love dies or leaves them. Instead of it going away or lessening, I think it was there from the moment she woke until the moment she went to sleep at night. Nightmares. Terrible. Shocking nightmares. She was terrified to sleep. She stopped taking all her anti-depressants and she spiralled downwards. She got so bad that she wouldn't get out of the bed.

With the stress and hurt of it all, she also suffered severe migraines and jaw pain. We thought they were a separate illness. We found her temporal muscles were swollen to twice their size from clenching her jaw at night. She was full of absolute anger—so angry. I've never seen anyone so angry; she was almost ready to explode all the time.

She felt this person that she'd split up from had destroyed her life, totally taken away the opportunity for her to have children, taken away from her the opportunity to have a home.

The headaches were so severe that she was taking prescription tablets. She was taking even more tablets trying to treat the headache, and it just wasn't working. She just laid there and this went on for weeks and weeks.

After the suicide attempt, we had people from the crisis centre coming out every day for two weeks. They assess you, you see the psychiatrist, they give you some information, and that's the end of it. There's no more they can do.

Unless that person wants to go and seek help, no one can help them.

You can, as a carer, have all these tactics to get them help, but unless they want to go, you can't do anything. Everyone just says to you, "Just leave her there. Just leave her in her own corner, and hopefully she'll want to see someone eventually."

Belinda was scared and afraid. She had paranoia, anxiety, everything just kept getting worse, absolutely worse and worse until I felt desperate, absolutely desperate.

I'd wake up in the morning sometimes afraid because she used to have such awful nights. I had to watch her medicine.

How did you manage to take care of yourself during that stage?

I used to tell myself that I couldn't let anything happen to me, because there was nowhere else for her; no one else would understand what she was going through.

I deprived myself. I didn't go anywhere or do anything. I was afraid to leave the house. I would hurry home. I had to quit my job for a while because there were days I couldn't go to work; she was so mentally ill and in physical pain. Every time the headache pain was removed I'd see this person so relieved and normal, but she would soon be back to the depressed anxious one.

At what point did you begin to get an understanding of what was going on with Belinda?

Probably, nearly a year after it started. I didn't know where to go. A psychiatrist actually rejected helping her, because she'd been there and they couldn't see any improvement after months. That was at her really low level.

That is when she had attempted the suicide, and she was ready to go back and get help. She was really ready to finally accept someone that could help her, and the day she went back there, they said, "We can't help you anymore." It knocked her socks off, and that's when she refused to get help from anybody at all.

Chapter 11: *"Love & Time the Healer" - A Mum's Journey with her Daughter*

I spent a lot of time on the internet. I'd try and find things that she could read that might be self-help, answers to her questions; I spent hours, hours and hours. What she was doing was letting me search.

Belinda actually told someone that if Mum couldn't save her, no one could.
What she was doing locking herself away, was healing, slowly. Time is the great healer.
She knew that my love for her was enough that I would search for things to help her. If I stopped, she would think, 'Oh, no one can help me now.'

How did you actually find the person that helped you? What made a difference?

I read about a hypnotherapist in the local paper. I managed to get Belinda to go to a lady who does hypnotherapy. I think Belinda was so desperate, she wanted the pills, someone to heal her, because she couldn't heal herself. I think in her mind, this lady was actually going to hypnotise her, like you see on television?

Belinda thought it would help her to see a clearer view on feeling happy again. When she got there, the lady who did the hypnotherapy was more on relaxation and thinking, using your mind to go to nice places. It wasn't anything like she thought. The hypnotist was helping her to help herself, and she couldn't understand that. She wanted the lady to do it all for her, like magic. We spent a very intense time there, and this woman was brilliant. Watching her work made me see a lot more, because I was allowed to sit in.

I actually saw how bad Belinda's thinking was. This lady described a forest, she was walking into a forest, and what did she see? This is when she got her to close her eyes and try to relax. Belinda saw a burnt forest, all burnt. Then she asked Belinda about a flower, and what did she see? She saw a drawing that a child would do. Everything was not real in her mind.

Also, Belinda didn't cope when the lady was describing an orange colour to her. All of a sudden Belinda said, "Stop it, stop it! I can't look at that colour anymore!" And she said to Belinda, "Well, what colour do you like?" Belinda said, "Maybe blue?"

At the end of the session, which went for two hours, I was really drained, and the lady actually had a few tears because Belinda was so flat, so negative, totally negative, all the time, about everything.

This lady said to me that she didn't think that we might be able to help her or save her.
I said, "Well, that's not going to happen. We're going to."

This lady was so distressed over the state of mind Belinda was in that she actually rang her sister and managed to get an appointment for Belinda to go and see her. Her sister does counselling for people like Belinda, and is very successful, she's very sought after.

The day that Belinda was supposed to go, an hour before, she said she didn't want to go.
I asked her if she would please go because this lady could help her, because she's been in the same place Belinda's been. I believed that only someone who has been in that place can connect with a person going through this.

I had to keep her going, to get through this terrible time, to a point where she could see a bit of light at the end of the tunnel and want to do things.

Before the appointment, she said, "I'm not going" which actually caused me to lose my temper.
I broke. I said, "You're ruining my life, taking over; I've got no happiness, nothing."

Then all of a sudden I saw the look of horror on her face, and I realised I might have done the worst thing ever. I said I was sorry; I didn't mean to hurt her, but I just didn't handle it any more because this lady was going to be the person that was going to start her on the right track and start to give her a bit of a life. I felt as though I'd be able to have a better life, without the drama. For that hope to be rejected was just too much for me.

Chapter 11: *"Love & Time the Healer" - A Mum's Journey with her Daughter*

What was the turning point for you?

I rang this lady to tell her that we weren't coming to the appointment, and she spent an hour with me on the phone, and she was the only person I've ever spoken to that really helped me.

That was the turning point; and that was the day I understood.

It opened my eyes up. I understood then what Belinda was actually going through.
When you actually understand what they're going through, it can appear hopeless for you, too.
I thought if this is happening in her mind and her body, where is it all going to end?

What this lady actually said to me was "I've got to step back and let Belinda decide what she wants to do with her life". I didn't want Belinda to stay locked away forever. Only Belinda can decide.

Belinda had to make that decision.
Yes. You end up their maid, otherwise.

What is the most important advice that anyone has ever given you on this journey?

This lady's advice, which I followed, is the best thing I did. I had done everything humanly possible.

I actually had a plan for every time one failed, I'd have another one. I was actually searching for the next plan when I got that advice. The advice she gave me was to step back. She said that I can't put her in cotton wool for the rest of her life. She has to be able to make the decision to live or die. Belinda is a strong girl.
Not long after that a friend of Belinda's came around unannounced. Belinda refused to see anyone and had a panic attack if she thought they were coming. The friend who came was an old friend, and she just turned up one day. She had pretty bad problems of her own with a marriage break-up and three kids. Belinda wanted to help her, and put her own problems aside.

Tracey Stranger

I also found Belinda watching the Victorian bush fires on television. She was in tears. She was starting to see the real world again. Belinda went and stayed with her girlfriend which was amazing to me, absolutely amazing. When she came home, her headache was pretty bad for a few days. Then a few weeks later, Belinda told me she was planning to move out and get a place of her own.

How does that make you feel?

Over the moon. Absolutely, Over the Moon. It's a big job, being a carer.

A lot of people don't realise, even though I have a job now, I can apply to get fifty dollars a week for carer's money. If your husband doesn't have a good job and you're struggling, you can actually get paid to be a carer for the person that you're caring for. At first when I went back to work, I rang them to tell them that I was working again, they told me it is a tax-free fifty dollars.

I thought to myself, 'I bloody earn it.' It keeps people like Belinda out of institutions. It is a help. I am sure there are a lot of people who get nothing because they don't know. Unless you ask for it, and put in an application, and find out about it, you won't know.

Belinda also had a disability pension. I found the people at Centrelink very caring and understanding. Belinda's doctor, she has a lot of faith in her, has been a very good support to Belinda; she always gives her a lot of time. She's very down to earth.

One time when I went to the doctor's with her, and I asked the doctor to talk and get Belinda to say she needs guidance, like from a psychiatrist or a counsellor, the doctor looked at me and she said, "You can lead a horse to water, but you can't make it drink." I was so frustrated that no one could help me to get her to counselling.
Now Belinda says she is going to go and see this hypnotherapist lady once she is in her own place.

Chapter 11: *"Love & Time the Healer" - A Mum's Journey with her Daughter*

That's a huge, huge step for Belinda

Yes. The place Belinda has got is an old place; so she can see things she can do to make it look nice, like painting and fixing it up. She is already thinking what plants she can put there. She wants to depend on herself, get her life back. To me, that is just fantastic. We've got through one of the worst years of my life. We are now stepping over a point where people, psychiatrists, people that have helped have all said things to me like, "You might not be able to save her." But, you know, you can't look at it like that.

You've got to go and take every step you can, right 'til the day either you may lose 'em, or, you see them coming back, and get their life back.

We've still got a lot of work to do because of these other health problems. I think that she can respect herself because she fought through the worst kind of depression you can have and she's now fighting her way back.

What helped you most get through that period?

For me, love. And I never gave up. There is also something within her that's pushed her along every day to keep going. Incredible given all the pain she's been in. Something inside me told me that Belinda would fight it through and move forward. I trusted my instinct. I was positive, always positive. Always turning the miserable thoughts into more positive thoughts. No matter what she came out with, I always found a way to turn my thoughts around.

Belinda didn't agree with me, but I did it anyway. I'll always say "You'll get rid of this pain one day. We've just got to find the answer." In the end, I told her that I'd done all I could and that she would have to try and start to help herself a little. Belinda did start to help herself.

There isn't anyone out there. You can ring counsel offices, where they'll make you an appointment. If the person that you're caring for won't go, they just stay, you almost beg them to come to your house. I was upset and desperately looking through the phone book.

Who can I ring?

Where can I get help?

Who can help me?

You think someone can come to your house and talk to them and help you, help them to understand what's actually going on. They say, "Oh, you're suffering depression." A lot of people don't sit and take the time to actually tell them what's happened to them.

A lot of people in the early stages of depression don't even know they're depressed. They just don't feel like they want to go to work; they don't feel like they want to do the housework or anything; they don't want to go anywhere.

Then it spirals into something more severe, if it's not caught in time.

What have been some of the most important things for you to keep yourself sane?

A very supportive and understanding husband. He was always there for me and didn't say too much. When the days were really bad, and he knew that I was going through a really bad time, he was supportive. My husband sleeps from two until ten at night, because he works night shift. It helped me that he wasn't taking my time away from the task of looking after Belinda.

In the mornings I got to spend time with him. We always made time on the weekend to go out to lunch or something. Visit friends. Talk to your family about your problems. There were only a couple of people I talked openly to at the time. I have come through this a lot stronger and I am able to get up and face every day now no matter what. I was continually looking for answers and finding understanding.

It was like living with a foreigner, a total stranger. I felt like she'd been possessed. I would think, "I've lost my daughter." I said to her one day, "I want this person to leave, and I want my daughter to come back."

You can't compare ill people with other ill people, because they're in their own world of torment. Sometimes mental illness can be far worse than actual physical illness, because your mind can control everything that you do. It controls your body; it controls your pain; it controls your emotions. Your mind is the one thing I think that can fix most things.

You can be in a really difficult situation. Some people sit back and laugh, and go, "Aah, How did I get myself into this?" which is probably what I would do.

Whereas Belinda would sit back and think it was the end of the world, and look at the total negative.
"Oh, what's happened? My whole life is ruined because of this. I'll never get over it." And spiral downwards, whereas I'll think, 'Oh, well, shit happens,' and try to get out of it.

What is important for family and friends to understand when you know someone who is depressed?

- The carer for someone with mental illness has to be thick skinned.
- You can't take the nasty comments to heart, because they don't mean it.
- They're hurting themselves so they lash out at everything around them. Belinda really wanted to be left alone in her own misery.
- They won't change before they're ready.
- You can't push them out the door.
- You've just got to give them the options, the time.
- Belinda started to do some things for herself.
- I always said, "You don't have to hurry. You've just got to take a little step at a time."
- I would say "One day when you wake up, you'll start to feel a bit better."
- Belinda did tell me that she was starting to feel a bit better.

Are there any final thoughts that you want to mention to help prevent others going into that downward spiral?

- I think the right counselling, early.
- If you went and saw one and you weren't happy, go immediately to find another. Not all personalities click.
- I think mental guidance in your thoughts, and direction, by a counsellor that can actually tell you things you can do to make

yourself feel better, and will share your problems and give you some advice. Someone that can be almost like sitting and talking to a friend.

- I always tell Belinda that the good times we've had far outweigh this experience. Really, it does.

It doesn't make sense that you've gone through this torment. Belinda growing up as a little girl, she always made me laugh. If anything was going to happen, it would happen to her. She could laugh about it in those days.

Belinda has been a good friend to me, and a good daughter; she has always been there if I needed her. Never missed my birthday, always came and did something with me on my birthday. I've enjoyed her being, and if I have to put up with some downside to being a parent, well, so be it, because I want to get the happy times back. I wanted my daughter back.

Now I am over the moon. We are heading in the right direction. Love and time are the healer.

Thank you so much for sharing your experience and it is so good Belinda is taking her own steps back into the world, with the help of her friend and her family.

IN SUMMARY

- Gain Understanding – I hope this book has given you a broader understanding of stress before it leads to greater severity. There is a rich resource guide also in this book. Talking to friends and family, a friendly ear anywhere is invaluable. Everyone has experienced some degree of stress in their life.
- Everyone's experience is unique. Listen with two ears. Be sincere, loving and ask: "How can I help you"? (Don't tell.)
- Find the Solution that's Right for Them. Never give up. If you are not happy with one doctor or therapist, find one that has got answers for you. Use this extensive resource guide to find a natural health practitioner in your area.
- Kindness – Be Kind to Yourself, you deserve it. Being a carer can be very tough work.

- Love –You are not your behaviour, your actions, your beliefs, your thoughts or your emotions. I love you, the heart of you. Let's work together to overcome the imbalance.
- Compassion – a deep awareness of the suffering of another, in a non-judgemental way.
- Human nature is naturally loving, kind and gentle.

"People who remain calm and open-minded, motivated by compassion are mentally free of anxiety and physically healthy. At a time when people are so conscious of maintaining their physical health by controlling their diets, exercising and so forth, it makes sense to try to cultivate the corresponding positive mental attitudes too."
Dalai Lama

DAILY ABC to Overcome Stress

1. ACCEPT the situation – It is what it is, now look for a positive practical solution. Accept your situation and share it with a friend, lighten your load, be honest and lovingly support yourself. Don't be the judge or dictator. Offer support and guidance.
2. BREATHE – Take a deep breath, Lighten the load on your shoulders, Keep breathing deeply. Oxygen is Life. Believe in yourself and Trust yourself.
3. CHANGE – Change your course of action. Do something different

DAILY MINDFULNESS

There is always a solution. LOVE will find a way.

Practise love and compassion to fellow sentient beings on a daily basis. Sometimes we are not in control of our actions and behaviours. May LOVE prevail and bring HOPE and PEACE.

I see the love in all no matter what their actions are.

Chapter 12:

Your Practical Day-to-Day Plan

Chapter 12:

Your Practical Day-to-Day Plan

In my own experience and helping others no matter what level of stress we experience, a daily plan is a key to coping with stress. Plan Your Work and Work Your Plan were wise words from my training manager in my early working years. That's all good and well, but "What if things don't go according to my plan?!"

KISS – Keep It Simple Stupid. That's the KISS principle. And that's true too.

What sort of plan and how simple to be most affective? Time appears to be getting faster, we seem to fit more into one day than we used to in one week. (Consciousness is evolving and accelerating so time and space are changing rapidly.)

If you get excited, and you are on a roll because you are getting a lot done, give yourself a pat on the back. Well Done! Do not pile more work on and overload yourself, take a deep breath first, and be gentle on yourself. Well Done for achieving MORE than what you set out. You don't have to keep proving more to yourself. (What is the monkey chatter of thoughts in your head telling you? Take notice.)

Some days fly like clockwork and you can have a magical day. The next day it may seem like every corner you turn is a road block and you hit a brick wall or an obstacle.

Take one step at a time. Take one day at a time. Each day is a new day.

Does this task really, really, really need to get done today?

Maybe you've never asked yourself that question. Maybe it can wait until tomorrow. Give yourself the space and stillness to realistically prioritise tasks.

Chapter 12: *Your Practical Day-toDay Plan*

Continually check in with yourself. When something unexpected lands on your lap, or on your desk, ask yourself a question.

Does this task really, really, really need to get done today?

Take a Deep Breath, Pause, Give Yourself time to REALISTICALLY assess the situation.

Now doesn't that feel better?

BRICK WALLS ARE BLESSINGS

How to learn from your greatest blows in life. Apply the ABC.
1. Accept the situation. What has happened, has happened. Let the dust settle.
2. Breathe Deeply. Take a few more deep breaths. Have some quiet time to absorb the change.
3. Control the situation. Take control by gathering information on potential options so you can make an informed decision and change the course of action. Look for a positive solution.

Here is a Practical Day to Day Plan. Using the ABC to Overcome Stress Naturally. You may wish to photocopy the page and work to your plan.

Remember KISS.

		Yes I did It! Give yourself a ✔	Your Notes What I learnt AND What I will do differently
On Waking Up EVERY MORNING	**A – Accept yourself, I am ok** **A – Ask and You Shall Receive** (in a still moment) **B – BREATHE – TAKE 3 DEEP BREATHS** Focus on the breath, TAKE 3 MORE DEEP BREATHS. Build up to 10 minutes each morn. **B – Balance – TAKE 3 DEEP BREATHS** **C – Change your Perception** • I am grateful for everything in my life • I am still and calm • I see the good in all		
6am – 9am 3 hours	**It is so IMPORTANT to start the DAY in a HEALTHY POSITIVE WAY** Create TIME to have a Simple Healthy Nourishing Breakfast: Protein, Fibre, Starch, Fruit. i.e. Eggs, Avocado, Tomato, Banana Protein –helps mental alertness & mental energy: Salmon, sardines chicken, turkey, lean red meat, oysters, crab • **SMILE – GENUINELY TO A STRANGER** Brighten up your day and somebody else's • Go for a walk • Go for a workout or swim • Exercise, Yoga, Be Creative		
9am – 12 midday 3 hours	**MINDFULNESS** 3 Deep Breaths – REGULARLY Throughout the whole day... **REMEMBER TO BE MINDFUL** Start to Notice Your Thoughts DON'T ATTACH TO THEM – JUST NOTICE **I WILL FOCUS and achieve my goal today. Prioritise, Prioritise, Prioritise.** Not everything is Urgent. Really! **BREATHE, BREATHE, BREATHE (Deeply)**		

Chapter 12:   *Your Practical Day-toDay Plan*

		Yes I did It! Give yourself a ✔	Your Notes What I learnt AND What I will do differently
12 – 1pm 1 hour	**CREATE 15 mins for lunch (at least).** Take time to sit down and eat your lunch – even if it is only 15 minutes. Take time out to eat. Time out for you. **Black Coffee & Dark Chocolate are rich in antioxidants and can boost your day.**		
1pm-4pm 3 hours	**Keep FOCUSSED on your task for today.** If there are distractions PRIORITISE. Eat An Apple a Day! Or some grapes or nuts.		
5pm – 7pm 2 hours	**Make time to have a healthy meal.** Organic hormone antibiotic free meat & chicken, Lean red meat. Talk to family, children, friends, share and care.		
7pm – 10pm 3 hrs	Apricots – antioxidants, iron, potassium Also help induce sleep and relaxation.		
BEDTIME	**Plan a Healthy 8 hour deep sleep to replenish.** Lie Down and TAKE 3 DEEP BREATHS, Relax, Balance. Acknowledge Yourself for achieving your goal. Give Thanks for the good in your life and send love to yourself and those you love. Be Grateful. Say at least one thing you are grateful for before you go to sleep each night.		

REMEMBER THE ABC OF OVERCOMING STRESS NATURALLY

A	B	C
Accept the situation	Breathe Deeply	Change your Perception
Acknowledge you are out of balance	Balance – seek balance	Change your Thoughts
Ask and Ye shall Receive	Be calm	Change your Beliefs
Ask "How can I?" Questions	Be still	Change your Actions
Allow yourself to rest, pause, take a deep breath	Be Peaceful Be Kind to Yourself	Change your Attitude to one of Gratitude
Act Now	Believe in yourself	Control the situation. Take control.

A FEW MORE TIPS FOR A STRESS FREE DAY

1. Dealing with The Internal Judge
2. Dealing with Persistent Emotions
3. Power Questions for Passion and Meaning

1. Dealing with The Internal Judge

The internal judge is the continual voice in your head that is giving you a hard time. Something is not right.

- Are you judging yourself?
- Get to know that internal judge?
- What is its story?
- Give it a personality

Be Mindful of this judge and simply become the witness to the judgemental conversation. You will recognise the conversation. You have heard it over and over and over again. Haven't you?
You are not your thoughts.

The next step to take is:

- Give thanks to your internal judge.
- Tell it "I no longer need your help to judge me and make me wrong".
- I do the best I can every day. Everything I do is perfect in every way. What I don't get done today, I can choose to get done on another day, and that's ok.
- I set you free. Now I am free.

www.HowToOvercomeStressNaturally.com

2. Dealing with persistent emotions use this ABC process to resolve the issue.

Step 1: Ask yourself these 4 questions:
1. Describe the emotion / feeling & write this down.
2. If you could give it a colour, what colour would it be?
3. If you could give it a shape, what shape would it be?
4. How dense on a scale of 1-10 is this?

This will objectify the situation. You start to separate from the emotion.

Step 2: Breathe and Detach
This emotion is not who you are. You are aware of the emotion. You are the one who is AWARE. You are not the emotion. Visualise this emotion floating above you, encased in a balloon, separate from you. This emotion inside the balloon is floating far away from you now.

Step 3: Cut the string and Release
Release this balloon, cut the string, let the balloon and those unwanted emotions drift far away. Take 3 Deep breaths. Focus on your heart. With each breath, fill yourself with peace and calm and love.

Say repeatedly:

I am calm, I am still, I am at peace.
I am calm, I am still, I am at peace.
I am Love, I am Love, I am Love.

Feed Yourself Positive Food for Thought.
Feed Yourself Positive Thoughts for Food.

Continue Breathing Deeply. Your heart is now clear of unwanted emotions and replaced with calm, peace and love. Notice how simple that is to do. You can do this whenever you need to. It's as simple as ABC. It really is.

3. Ask Yourself these Power Questions

How can I do what I love to do and make money?
How can I do what I love to do and help others?
How can I do what I love to do and help others make money?
How can I help others?
- You may have a solution to their problem
- You may be able to lift their spirit
- You may be able to bring friendship, fun and laughter into their life
- You may bring knowledge they are seeking
- You may have skills they need
- You may bring hope, encouragement and motivation
- You may bring them love.

How can I help the environment?
- You may join a group you are passionate about
- You may create a group with a common cause
- You may offer your skills, love and passion

Talk to a friend – choose someone who can help you find positive solutions.

Remember to talk to your local friendly and knowledgable Naturopath at Natural Health Food stores and Pharmacies.

If it is your passionate intention to find a positive solution YOU WILL. Energy follows Awareness. Whatever you focus on will grow in energy and momentum.

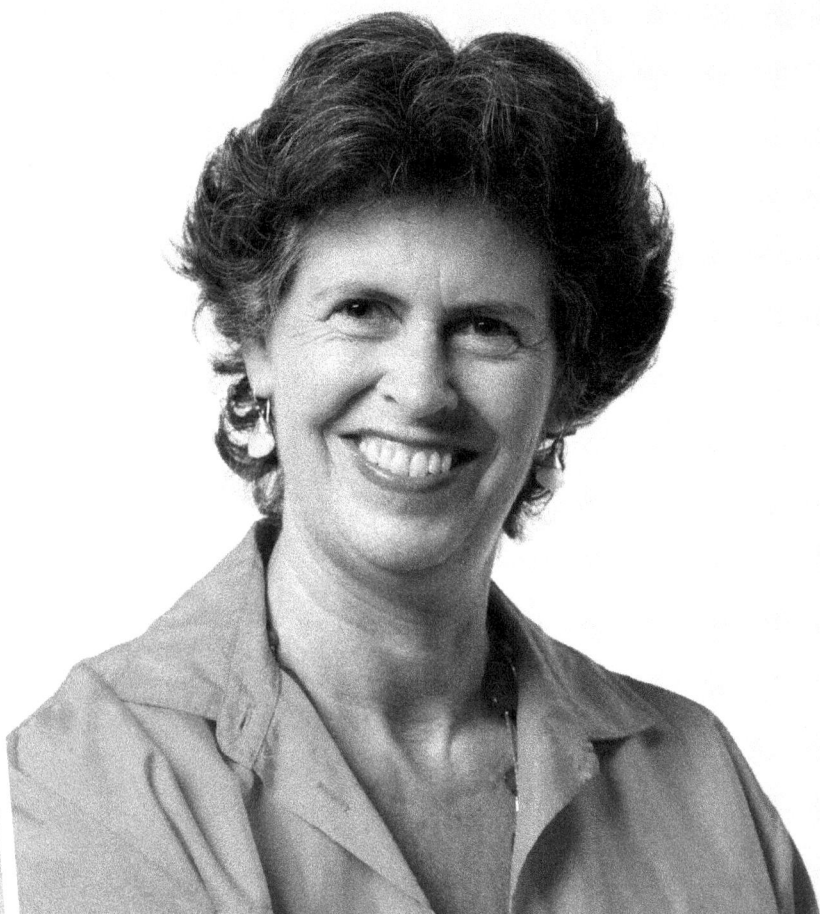

Chapter 13:

Final Note from the Author

Chapter 13:

Final Note from the Author

I have spoken to leaders in their field of western medicine and natural medicine and I have spoken to everyday people. Each and every one are stars in their own life achievements. Just as you are a star in your own life achievement.

- You are in charge of your life, your thoughts and your beliefs.
- Create each day with passion and enthusiasm.
- Take a small step each day, let your journey unfold.
- Be open to new opportunities, new ideas, new connections, meeting new people.
- Listen to your intuition, your inner wisdom. Trust your inner knowing.
- In these times of economic change it is ever more important to look after your health – physical, mental & emotional.

You have learnt in this book the power of the Mind, how it can influence your thoughts and moods.

You have also learnt the powerful effect food has on mood and our physical wellbeing.

It makes good sense to make wise choices regarding what you think and what you eat.

This book can help you make wise choices regarding your health – physical, mental and emotional.

I think the best (always aiming for a win-win) and most of the time – it happens.

I have a friend who often thinks the worst and "what if" and guess what – most of the time it happens.

The choice is yours. You can choose your thoughts. You can break an unhealthy habit. The choice is yours.

To change direction and start creating a new and richer life for you, begin step by step, one day at a time.

Use the Practical Day-To-Day Plan in this book to get you started.

Chapter 13: *Final Note from the Author*

Photocopy the Mindfulness Activities, Power Actions and Meditations and Contemplations at the end of each chapter and use them daily. Stick them on your bedroom, study, kitchen wall to remind you.
There are more practical tools and templates at my website
www.HowToOvercomeStressNaturally.com

Take Control of Your Mental, Emotional and Physical Health right now. You are more powerful than you can imagine. In fact, dare to dream, dare to imagine, be true to yourself and think and act for the good of all.

Let Go of your chaotic thoughts, which will influence how you feel so it will be easier to let go of negative emotions and Let Go of structures that no longer serve you.

Build new creative beliefs and thoughts with a focused goal in mind. Grow love and compassion for yourself and all of humanity and Build new structures that serve you, your family, your community and humanity.

Choose to live from Love and Abundance rather than scarcity and fear. I do.

Choose to live a Prosperous Life so you can help others do the same. That's my goal.

Hang out with people who believe in you and fly together.
Most of all enjoy the choices you make. Remember you can change your world. I know you can. Do you?

Come visit my website **www.HowToOvercomeStressNaturally.com** for:

- Inspirational Daily Quotes – to help you change your Mindset
- Daily Mindfulness Activities
- Daily Meditations / Contemplations
- Day-To-Day Template – to help you plan your day to day to build your new future
- Weekly Template – to help you the steps to achieve your goals, step by step
- To Write your Story of Success "How You Overcome Stress Naturally" using any of these tools
- To claim your free DVD on the Mayan Calendar 2012 – presented by Ian Xel Lungold. Time is speeding up, our environment is changing – it's called evolution. A practical no-nonsense informative DVD, supported by real events in history. Recommended for all ages.

SOME SUGGESTED GROUPS TO JOIN & BOOKS TO READ

Astronomical Society of Australia
http://www.astronomy.org.au

Australian Astronomy is an official web site of the Astronomical Society of Australia featuring extensive links to astronomical research, teaching, and public education facilities and activities in Australia. http://asa.astronomy.org.au/

2009 is International Year of Astronomy. The Universe is Yours to Discover. This marks the 400th anniversary of Galileo's first turning of a telescope towards the heavens.

The International Year of Astronomy (IYA) is an initiative of the International Astronomical Union, endorsed by the United Nations, to help the people of Earth realise their place in the Universe and to appreciate the beauty and wonder of the sky above.

Astronomical Association of Queensland
http://www.aaq.org.au/cms/

Astronomical Society of NSW
http://www.asnsw.com/

Astronomical Society of Victoria
http://www.asv.org.au/

Astronomical Society South Australia
http://www.assa.org.au/observing/welcome/

Western Australia's Astronomy and Space Science Community
http://www.astronomywa.net.au/

Australian Amateur Astronomy Societies and Groups in Australia
http://www.quasarastronomy.com.au/society.htm

Chapter 13: *Recommended Groups*

Dolphin Research Institute
http://www.dolphinresearch.org.au/   Victoria, Australia
Ph: 1300 130 949
To ensure the wellbeing of dolphins and the marine environment.

You can Adopt-A-Dolphin which is a wonderful gift for yourself or someone else and supports Dolphin Research.

Essential Health Australia Pty Ltd
http://www.essentialhealth.com.au
Everything essential for your health and wellbeing. Aromatherapy, Massage oils, Natural Soaps.

Expanding Energies
http://www.expandingenergies.com.au/
Meditation CD's for adults and children, The Art of Breathing CD, Workshops and Readings.

Inspirational Books
To Touch A Wild Dolphin – The Lives & Minds of the Dolphins of Monkey Mia
By Rachel Smolker

The Body is the Barometer of the Soul – So Be Your Own Doctor
By Annette Noontil

Reconnect with the Heart and Remember the Soul
Poems, Acronyms and Affirmations for Inspiration and Meditation
By Elizabeth Joy

Wings Back to Go Forward – Happiness Is Just A Breath Away
By Kawena (Gwen Gordon)

The Liver Cleansing Diet - By Dr Sandra Cabot

The Prophet - By Kahlil Gibran

The Little Prince - By Antoine De Saint-Exupéry

RESOURCE DIRECTORY
Australian Official bodies and Associations

beyondblue – The national depression initiative
http://www.beyondblue.org.au
INFOLINE: 1300-224-636

Hawthorn, Victoria

beyondblue is a national, independent, not-for-profit organisation devoted to increasing awareness and understanding of depression in the community. We do not have doctors, counsellors or health professionals available to respond to your specific difficulties. Unfortunately, we do not have the capacity to respond to urgent or personal requests for help or advice.

Black Dog Institute Australia
http://www.blackdoginstitute.org.au/index.cfm   Randwick, NSW
Director: Prof Gordon Parker
Phone: 02 9382 4530

The Black Dog Institute is a non-profit educational, research, clinical and community-oriented facility offering specialist expertise in mood disorders. The Institute is attached to the Prince of Wales Hospital and affiliated with the University of New South Wales.

DepressioNet – Resources to help you with depression
http://www.workingwell.org.au/depressionet-2.html

DepressioNet operates around the clock improving the mental health and well being of people impacted by mild to moderate depression through; the Information Service, which provides people with the right tools to locate information on resources, healthcare professionals, causes of depression and treatment options.

Post & Antenatal Depression Association Inc.
www.panda.org.au   North Fitzroy, Victoria
Ph: 1300 726 306
PANDA is a Victorian, not-for-profit, self-help organisation that was formed in 1985 to provide confidential information, support and referral

to anyone affected by post and antenatal mood disorders, including partners and extended family members. PANDA also produces and distributes accurate information about post and antenatal mood disorders to health professionals and the wider community.

Mental Health Foundation Australia

http://www.mentalhealthvic.org.au/   Richmond, Victoria
Ph: 03 9427 0406

The Mental Health Foundation of Australia (Victoria) membership encompasses people living with mental illness, family members, carers and friends, professionals from many fields, mental health service providers and interested members of the general public.

Multicultural Mental Health Australia

http://www.mmha.org.au
Provides national leadership in building greater awareness of mental health and suicide prevention amongst Australians from culturally and linguistically diverse backgrounds.

Mental Health Council of Australia

http://www.mhca.org.au/

Established in 1997, the Mental Health Council of Australia (MHCA) is the peak, national non-government organisation representing and promoting the interests of the Australian mental health sector, committed to achieving better mental health for all Australians.

MHCA Members include national organisations representing consumers, carers, special needs groups, clinical service providers, public and private mental health service providers, researchers and state/territory community mental health peak bodies.

ACOSS – Australian Council of Social Services

http://www.acoss.org.au
The Australian Council of Social Service (ACOSS) is the peak council of the community services and welfare sector. Established in 1956, ACOSS is the national voice for the needs of people affected by poverty and inequality.

Mental Health Associations are in each state of Australia

SANE Australia

http://www.sane.org/
HELP LINE: 1800 187 263

SANE Australia is a national charity working for a better life for people affected by mental illness.

The SANE Mind and Body Initiative focuses on treatment and support for the whole person: promoting better physical health for people with a mental illness, and better mental health for people with physical health conditions.

LifeLine

http://www.lifeline.org.au/
Phone: 13 11 14

Lifeline was founded in 1963 by the late Reverend Dr Sir Alan Walker, after he received a call by a distressed man, who three days later took his own life. Determined not to let loneliness, isolation or anxiety be the cause of other deaths, Sir Alan launched a crisis line, which operated out of the Methodist Central Mission in Sydney. Lifeline's services now operate from 60 locations nationally, with a presence in every State and Territory within Australia.

Stress Down 24/7 (24th July)

http://www.stressdown.org.au

Stress Down Day encourages everyone to have fun and participate in stress reducing activities, but it's important to remember that stress is a serious issue affecting many of us.

Mensline Australia

http://www.menslineaus.org.au/
Phone: 1300 78 99 78

Our Vision is to empower Australian men to actively participate in building and sustaining healthy personal relationships that support healthy families, workplaces and communities.

Chapter 13: *Resource Directory*

Youth Help

Headspace – Australia's National Youth Mental Health Foundation
http://www.headspace.org.au/   Sunshine, Victoria
Phone: 03 9349 5804

If you or someone you know is going through a tough time, we can help with useful information, where to get help, what to expect when you get there, stories from others and events you can attend. There are 30 youth friendly health services located across Australia for young people 12 – 25 and their families.

GROW
http://www.grow.net.au/   Holland Park, Qld
Ph: 07 3397 7629

GROW is a community of persons working towards mental health through mutual help and a 12 step program of recovery. Small groups of people who have experienced depression, anxiety or other mental or emotional distress, come together on a weekly basis to help each other deal with the challenges of life. Some people come to GROW while struggling with the loss of a job, a loved one or a relationship.

Kids Helpline
http://www.kidshelp.com.au   Milton, Qld
HELP LINE: 1800 551 800 – 24 hour telephone FREE call, and online counselling.

Kids Help Line is Australia's only free, confidential and anonymous, telephone and online counselling service specifically for young people aged between 5 and 25.

Youthbeyondblue
http://www.youthbeyondblue.com/

Youthbeyondblue's all about getting the message out there that it's okay to talk about depression, and to encourage young people and their family and friends to get help when it's needed.

One in five young Australians experience depression each year, and more than half of those aren't getting the professional help they need to get through it.

Orygen Youth Health

www.orygen.org.au

Phone: 03 9342 2800   Parkville, Victoria

At Orygen Youth Health we are working to ensure that young people are able to access high quality mental health and drug and alcohol services provided in friendly, accessible environments.

Headroom

http://www.headroom.net.au/   South Australia

Headroom is a South Australian mental health promotion project managed by the Division of Mental Health, Women's and Children's Hospital which is part of the Children Youth and Women's Health Service. The Headroom project is supported on a state-wide level by Southern CAMHS, Flinders Medical Centre.

This website aims to inform young people, their caregivers and service providers about positive mental health. For Young people aged 12 -18 in the Lounge, young people aged 6-12 years in the Cubby House, parents and friends in the Family Room and Service providers and professionals in the Kitchen.

Sunrise Foundation

http://www.sunrisefoundation.org.au/   Melbourne, Victoria

Phone: 03 8346 8220

The Sunrise Foundation is a non profit organisation created to develop and deliver purpose built preventative education programs addressing depression for young people aged between 12-24 years. Education provider.

Inspire Foundation

http://www.inspire.org.au/

Phone: 02 8585 9300   Rozelle, NSW

The Inspire Foundation was established in 1996 in direct response to Australia's then escalating rates of youth suicide. We combine technology with the direct involvement of young people to deliver innovative and practical online programs that prevent youth suicide and improve young people's mental health and wellbeing. Our mission is to help millions of young people lead happier lives.

Chapter 13:   *Resource Directory*

The Jean Hailes Foundation for Women's Health
http://www.healthforwomen.org.au   Clayton, Victoria
Toll Free: 1800 151 441

Information on health for women.

Australian Depression Institute
http://adi.net.au/   Maleny, Queensland
Phone: 61 7 5494 2900

2 day Intensive Program, 9 day Integration, 16-28 Retreat Immersion Program. The Australian Depression Institute has spent the last 5 years committed to achieving one goal: to help individuals beat depression and anxiety. Drug free and fully supported by many Doctors, psychologists and leading health professionals our simple yet revolutionary approach both changes and saves lives.

Fountainhead Organic Health Retreat
(Linked with Australian Depression Institute.)
http://www.fountainhead.com.au   Maleny, Queensland
Phone: 61 (07) 5494 3495

Since we opened our doors, just over six years ago, we have served over 2000 Guests who needed help with fitness, a Pamper, a Juice Detox or had a serious health issue to deal with. We operate within a working Organic farm in Maleny (right next to the Glasshouse Mountains) Queensland, one of the most beautiful spots in Australia.

Back from the Brink Book – Australians tell their stories of Overcoming Depression
by Graeme Cowan
http://www.iambackfromthebrink.com/
Extensive National & International Resource Section

The Gawler Foundation

www.gawler.org   Yarra Junction, Yarra Valley, Victoria

Phone: 03 5967-1730

The Gawler Foundation is committed to an integrated approach to health, healing and wellbeing that includes the body, emotions, mind and spirit. We call this integrative medicine. We believe that every person is worthy of great respect. We believe that while in our hearts each person has the same pure essence, each person does need to be treated as a unique individual. While we respect all valid forms of external treatment, we believe that true healing comes from within. Our deepest aspiration is to support each individual to seek their own inner truth, to realise it and to live by it.

Our residential programs are conducted in the beautiful foothills of the Yarra Valley at our purpose built site – The Yarra Valley Living Centre – at Yarra Junction.

The Lewis Institute For Health & Wellbeing

www.pathways2wellbeing.com.au   Prahran, Victoria

Phone: 61 3 9529 6094

In line with our purpose to enhance health and wellbeing we provide whole person education, programmes and services to the public and to health care practitioners. We also have an active research programme devoted to determining the evidence-base for integrative therapies. We hold courses, lectures and seminars. The people who lead our courses are carefully selected for their expertise and educational skills. They are from the disciplines of Medicine, Physiotherapy, Occupational Therapy, Psychology, Nutrition, Science and Yoga.

Chapter 13:   *Resource Directory*

The Quest for Life Centre
www.questforlife.com.au

Phone: +61 (02) 4883 6599   Bundanoon, NSW
Program enquiries and bookings 1300-941-488

The Quest for Life Foundation was established in 1990 by Petrea King to further her work. Since her recovery from leukaemia in 1984, Petrea has devoted her life to counselling people, facilitating support groups, running residential programs and lecturing widely on health and healing.

Petrea and the work of Quest for Life is at Bundanoon in the beautiful Southern Highlands of NSW.
The Quest for Life Centre, is set in 9 tree filled acres, provides an oasis for time out and an ideal environment for reflection, healing and the learning of new and valuable life skills.

The Quest for Life Foundation provides a range of residential programs and services that encourage, empower and educate people living with cancer, neurological and other serious illnesses, or who are suffering from grief, stress or trauma and for those who care for them.

NEW ZEALAND

Mental Health Foundation of New Zealand
http://www.mentalhealth.org.nz
Go To"Resource & Information Service"

Phone:
Auckland   (09) 300 7010
Wellington   644-384-4002
Christchurch   (03) 366 6936

The Mental Health Foundation works towards creating a society free from discrimination, where all people enjoy positive mental health and well-being. Our work seeks to influence individuals, wh nau, organisations and communities to improve and sustain their mental health and reach their full potential.

Ours is a holistic approach that supports emotional and spiritual well-being and respects the importance of culture, equity, social justice and personal dignity.

The foundation is not a counselling or advice service, but we can point you in the right direction - just visit our Resource & Information Service.

Mental Health Commission
http://www.mhc.govt.nz/
Go To "Information resources"
New Zealand will be a nation where New Zealanders sustain their mental health and wellbeing, and when any one of us experience mental illness and/or addiction we are able to lead our recovery by participating in our communities and accessing high quality, responsive services.

About one in five adult New Zealanders experience mental health or addiction problems.
That makes mental health everyone's business.

USA

National Institute of Mental Health
http://www.nimh.nih.gov   Besthesda, MD, USA
Go To "Health & Outreach / Mental Health Topics"
Phone: 1-866-615-6464 (toll-free)

The largest scientific organisation in the world dedicated to research focused on the understanding, treatment, and prevention of mental disorders and the promotion of mental health.

American Institute of Stress
http://www.stress.org/   Yonkers, New York, USA
Phone: 914-963-1200

Dedicated to advancing our understanding of the role of stress in Health & Illness, the nature and importance of Mind-Body Relationships and how to utilise our vast innate potential for Self-Healing.

Chapter 13: *Resource Directory*

CANADA

Canadian Mental Health Association
http://www.cmha.ca/   Ottawa, Canada
Phone: 613-745-7750

The Canadian Mental Health Association is a nation-wide charitable organisation that promotes the mental health of all, and supports the resilience and recovery of people experiencing mental illness.

Mental Health Canada
http://www.mentalhealthcanada.com/   Ontario, Canada
Phone: (416) 652-9474

A national comprehensive directory of Psychiatrists, Psychologists, Psychoanalysts, Counsellors, and Psychotherapists searchable by professional designation, gender and location. Mental health professionals offer medical treatment and/or specialise in individual, couples, marital, family or group therapy.

INTEGRATIVE MEDICINE

Australasian Integrative Medicine Association (AIMA)
http://www.aima.net.au/index.jsp   South Melbourne, Victoria

Go To"Practitioners"to find an integrative medicine health professional in your area.
Ph: (03) 8699 0582

Your Health
http://www.yourhealth.com.au/
Brighton (Victoria), Mermaid Beach (Qld), Manly (NSW), Sandy Bay (Tas)
Telephone: 61 (02) 9977 7888

Your Health centres are medical practices providing high quality Integrative Medicine services to achieve the best possible health outcomes.

USA

International College of Integrative Medicine
http://www.icimed.com/   Bluffton, Ohio, USA
Go To "Find a Practitioner" search by speciality or by zip code.
Ph: 866-464-5226 ICIM Toll Free OR 419-358-0273

American College for Advancement of Medicine (ACAM)
http://www.acamnet.org   Laguna Hills, California, USA
Go To "Resources / Physician + Link (Find a Doctor)"
Phone: 949-309-3520

A not-for-profit association dedicated to educating physicians and other health care professionals on the latest findings and emerging procedures in complementary, alternative and integrative (CAIM) medicine. ACAM enables members of the public to connect with physicians who take an integrative approach to patient care and empowers people with information about integrative medicine treatment options.

The American Association of Naturopathic Physicians
http://www.naturopathic.org   Washington, DC, USA
Go To "Find an ND"
Phone: 866-538-2267 toll-free OR 202-237-8150

Representing Naturopathic Doctors, Physicians Who Listen.

CANADA

Health Action Network Society
http://www.hans.org/   Burnaby, BC, Canada
Ph: 604 435 0512
Go To "Wellness Directory" for an extensive list of health practitioners in various modalities.

HANS (Health Action Network Society) is a charitable natural health resource. HANS provides information on preventive medicine and natural therapeutics through our website, a reference library, Health Action magazine, the HANS e-News, and regular educational and networking events. Our members are like-minded people of all backgrounds, lay and professional, who share an interest in a natural approach to health care.

Chapter 13: *Resource Directory*

NUTRITION & ENVIRONMENTAL MEDICINE

Australasian College Nutrition & Environmental Medicine (ACNEM)
http://www.acnem.org   Sandringham, Victoria
Go To "Products & Services / Referrals" - Find a Health Professional in your state, Australia & NZ.
Ph: +61 (03) 9597 0363

A non-profit organisation, funded from membership fees, subscriptions, courses and other programs, book sales and donations.

UK

British Society for Ecological Medicine (BSEM)
http://www.ecomed.org.uk/   London, UK
Go To "Find a Practitioner"
Ph: +44 207 100 7090

The BSEM promotes the study and good practice of allergy, environmental and nutritional medicine for the benefit of the public, and supports doctors who use the insights of ecological medicine to help patients.
If you are a patient looking for a practitioner of ecological medicine, you can find one on the Practitioners List.

USA

American Holistic Medical Association (AHMA)
http://www.holisticmedicine.org   Beachwood, Ohio
Go To "Public / Practitioner Finder"
Phone: (216) 292-6644

The AHMA was founded in 1978 to unite licensed physicians who practice holistic medicine. It is the oldest holistic medicine organisation of its kind, and many of today's national leaders in holistic medicine got their start as members of the AHMA. Since its first meeting in Denver, Colorado, the AHMA has continued to strive toward creating fellowship and collaboration among practitioners and those they work with - bringing an understanding of how the mind, the body and the spirit all have a part to play in healing.

The Institute for Functional Medicine

http://www.functionalmedicine.org/ Gig Harbour, WA, USA

Go To "Find FM Practitioner", including an extensive worldwide practitioner database
Phone: 800-228-0622 OR 253-858-4724

Our Mission is to serve the highest expression of individual health through widespread adoption of functional medicine as the standard of care.

Functional Medicine is patient-centred health care that addresses the unique interactions among genetic, environmental and lifestyle factors influencing both health and complex, chronic disease.

AYURVEDA

Australasian Ayurvedic Practitioners Association
Shanti Gowans – President
http://www.ayurvedapractitionersaustralia.com/
Ph: 07 5531 1141 Gold Coast, Queensland

Australasian Association of Ayurveda
Contact: Dr Krishna Kumar
Ph: 08 8366 6516 Ridleyton, South Australia

The Meditation Institute – Shanti Yoga™ – The Healing Path
http://www.shantiyoga.com.au/
Ph: +61 (07) 5531 0511 Southport, Queensland

The Meditation Institute boldly explores new frontiers and advances education, spiritual practices, healing and research for the expansion and wellbeing of mind-body and spirit as well as human consciousness through the teachings and programs of Shanti Gowans. Our services and products are inspirational aids created for the integration of mind, body, spirit and the environment.

Nirvana Organic-Eco-Retreat Sanctuary, consists of 70 hectares situated in dairy/rain-forest country, a complete retreat from the outside world, approximately 8kms from Beechmont, in Queensland, Australia.

Omyayush Holistic Health Centre

http://www.omayush.com.au/   Adelaide, South Australia
Phone 08 8272 1820

Ayurveda offers unique, long lasting and the most wonderful treatment for stress and stress related disorders through detoxification and rejuvenation programme. Treatment consists of abhyanga (traditional indian massage), swedan (medicated steam therapy) and shirodhara followed by lifestyle and dietary advice, herbal supplements (if necessary) and suggestions on practical meditation techniques.

Ayush Ayurveda Centre Melbourne

http://www.ayushayurved.com.au/vedic-beauty-care.html
Phone: +61 3 9401 5379   Epping, Victoria

Every treatment offered in Ayush Ayurveda Centre is structured according to each individual's constitution and need, commonly known as your body type by Dr. S. Chahal. With specific massages, detoxifying therapies and natural beauty care, be prepared to gift yourself a new life, surrender to the magical fingers of our specially trained Ayurvedic therapists and experience how they create a new person- bubbling with endless energy from within yourself.

Ayurve Beauty & Wellness Day Spa - 5,000 years of proven results
http://www.ayurveda.com.au

Tel: +61 (0)2 9279 3719   Sydney, New South Wales

Ayurve is a popular and the best day spa and holistic beauty, conveniently situated in the heart of the Sydney C.B.D for your convenience.

Heritage Healers Holistic Skin Care
http://www.heritagehealers.com.au
Phone: +61 (0)2 9905 2136   Brookvale, NSW

Immerse yourself in the healing world of Ayurveda - a sacred space where your mind, body, soul and skin are blissfully nurtured and united. We balance the body's diverse energies using your personal wildflower essence remedy and the ancient art of Ayurvedic energy work, known as Chakra Balancing. Your therapist works with the body's natural flow of energy to release stress, re-align and restore balance.

Trinity Health
http://www.trinityhealth.com.au   Melbourne, Victoria
Phone: Ph: +61   (03) 9687 4029 Dr. Sajimon George (Ayurvedic)
Ph: + 61 (03) 9478 8649   Raj Kothuru (Homeopathic)

Ayurveda and Homeopathy together is a treasure to all mankind; it offers us a gateway to health that is available to all those who truly seek it. We have combined the finest of Ayurvedic and Homeopathic practices and made it available affordably to everyone in search of a healthy life.

Yatan Holistic Ayurvedic Centre
http://www.yatan-ayur.com.au/index.htm
Ph: 1300 552 260 OR   (02) 9499 7164   Gordon, NSW

Prior to moving to Sydney and establishing YATAN Holistic Ayurvedic Centre in January 2000, Raman Das had a successful International Ayurvedic clinic in Kathmandu, Nepal, and also spent many years living and teaching Yoga at his ashram (Mahatyagi Seva Ashram) in Varanasi, India.

Walking On Clouds Wellness Centre
http://www.walkingonclouds.com.au
Ph: +61 (089) 218 8881   Perth, Western Australia

An Ayurvedic consultation consists of an in-depth analysis of your health, determining your own individual constitution, and examining any imbalances that may be present. We provide Corporate Massage

Chapter 13: *Resource Directory*

for a number of businesses in Perth's CBD. Our therapists come to your office and perform a back and shoulder table massage for members of your staff. The massage is a therapeutic massage and our therapists can incorporate healing with the massage.

Kids & Teens Treats are a terrific way to relieve the stress and tension that being in your teens can bring; so escape life and forget about your cares for a while. Remember how important you are!

NEW ZEALAND

The New Zealand Ayurvedic Association
http://www.ayurveda.org.nz/
Go To "Links/Member's Sites" to find Ayurvedic Practices in NZ.

The New Zealand Ayurvedic Association Inc., was formed in 2003 to support Ayurveda and Yoga students, schools, suppliers, practitioners and enthusiasts. The purpose of this website is to gather information on Ayurveda and on yoga; so that it can become an invaluable resource for all those interested in Ayurveda and yoga.

Planet Ayurveda. Wellness & Spa Centre
http://www.planetayurveda.co.nz   Mt Eden, Auckland
Tel: (09) 623 2651

Established in 1996 by Dr S. Ajit, to practice and teach Ayurveda in its totality aiming at prevention, cure and rejuvenation of the whole being keeping up with the original Ayurvedic philosophy, texts and values thus promoting a balanced holistic way of life.

INDIA

Kerala Ayurvedic Health Care
http://www.keralaayurvedichealthcare.com

A Traditional Ayurveda Panchakarma Centre situated at New Delhi and branches at Gurgaon Bindapur, Janak Puri and Trivandrum in Kerala, India.

USA

National Ayurvedic Medical Association

http://www.ayurveda-nama.org/   Santa Cruz, CA, USA
Ph: 1800 669 8914

Go To "Practitioner Directory" to find an Ayurvedic practitioner in your area.

The National Ayurvedic Medical Association is a national organisation representing the Ayurvedic profession in The United States of America. Its mission is to preserve, protect, improve and promote the philosophy, knowledge, science and practice of Ayurveda for the benefit of humanity.

Chopra Centre

http://www.chopra.com/ccwbwelcome.htm   Carlsbrad, CA, USA
Ph: 760 494 1600 OR 888 424 6772

Fulfilling a lifelong dream of creating a centre which focuses on enhancing health and nourishing the human spirit, Deepak Chopra, M.D. and David Simon M.D. opened The Chopra Centre For Wellbeing in 1996 in San Diego. Located in the midst of the world famous La Costa Resort & Spa, the Chopra Centre is an ideal place to heal, recharge and re-connect with your soul.
The Chopra Centre is a safe haven of non-judgment where travellers visit to reconnect with their unconditioned selves. Guests learn to cope with physical, emotional, and health related states of imbalance. Using the timeless wisdom of meditation, Ayurveda, and conscious communication, guests immerse themselves in the principles that Drs. Chopra & Simon have shared for decades.

UK

Ayurvedic Practitioners Association

http://www.apa.uk.com/   (Brighton, UK)
Go To "Find a Practitioner or Therapist" search by name or location
Ph: 01273 500 492

To facilitate the health, happiness and well-being of all, we manifest the truth of Ayurveda through unity and love.

Chapter 13:   *Resource Directory*

EUROPE

Ayurveda Institute of Europe
http://www.ayurvedainstitute.org/
Go To "Register of Therapists"

The Ayurveda Institute of Europe is a leading Institute that teaches ayurvedic courses such as ayurvedic body massage (abhyanga), ayurvedic face massage, ayurvedic back massage, ayurvedic foot massage, ayurvedic ear massage, ayurvedic head massage (shirobhyanga) as opposed to Indian head massage, shirodhara, advanced ayurvedic massage training, ayurvedic training-ayurvedic beauty facials, henna art, threading, nutrition, Ayurveda Diploma, reiki and meditation.

TRADITIONAL & CHINESE MEDICINE

The Australian Acupuncture and Chinese Medicine Association (AACMA)
http://www.acupuncture.org.au/
Go To "Click here to Find Practitioner" in your local suburb.

The Australian Acupuncture and Chinese Medicine Association Ltd (AACMA) is the leading national professional association of acupuncture and Traditional Chinese Medicine (TCM) practitioners.

Acupuncture and Traditional Chinese Medicine Resource
Go To "Find a Practitioner".
http://www.acupuncture.com.au/practitioner/search.html

The Australian Traditional Medicine Society (ATMS)
http://www.atms.com.au/
Ph: +61 (02) 9289 6809   Sydney, NSW
Go To "Find a Practitioner" in your local area or country.

The Australian Traditional-Medicine Society (ATMS) is Australia's largest professional association of complementary medicine practitioners, representing about 65% of the total complementary medicine profession.

CANADA

Traditional Chinese Medicine Association of British Columbia (TCMABC)
http://www.tcmabc.org/   Vancouver, Canada
Go To "Find a Practitioner"
Ph: 604 602 7550

The TCMABC exists for practitioners of TCM with the goal of supporting our members in the spirit of open-communication, & cooperation. Support comes in the form of representation, education, and increased public awareness to create a unified, successful, and healthy TCM practitioner community.

American Academy of Medical Acupuncture
http://www.medicalacupuncture.org/   El Segundo, California, USA
Go To "Find an Acupuncturist near you" by state or telephone area code.
Ph: (310) 364 0193

The purpose of the American Academy of Medical Acupuncture is to promote the integration of concepts from traditional and modern forms of acupuncture with Western medical training and thereby synthesize a more comprehensive approach to health care.

NATURAL THERAPY

Australian Natural Therapists Association (ANTA)
http://www.australiannaturaltherapistsassociation.com.au
Ph: 1800 817 577   Maroochydore, Queensland

Go To Practitioners: Find Health online, Search, Choosing a Therapist - to find one in your area

The Australian Natural Therapists Association Limited (ANTA) is the largest national democratic association of 'recognised professional' traditional medicine and natural therapy [Complementary Medicine] practitioners who work in the areas of health care and preventative medicine.

Chapter 13: *Resource Directory*

HeartMath Australasia

http://www.heartmath.com.au/   Sydney, Australia
Ph: 02 9412 2500
Go To "News & PR"

The HeartMath global network includes licensee companies in UK, Sweden, Netherlands, France, Korea, Australia/NZ and the global headquarters in USA.

Doc Lew Childre is the founder of HeartMath and a global authority on optimising human performance and personal effectiveness. In 1991 Doc founded the non-profit Institute of HeartMath (IHM) to research the effects of mental and emotional stress on the heart, brain and nervous system.

The Australian Breathwork Association

http://www.australianbreathworkassociation.org.au/
Tel: 02 9499 9895 0402 067024   Thornleigh, NSW
Go To "Find a Practitioner"

Breathwork is a tool for inner work using full, conscious, connected breathing, a technique that can provide resolution and clearing of issues, patterns and beliefs on a cellular level, spontaneous and organic beyond the mundane, a sacred, soulful experience.
Breathwork can be done as one-to-one sessions with a practitioner or in a group setting.

Institute of Heart Intelligence

http://www.breathwork.com.au/
Ph: +61 (03) 9739 8889   Melbourne, Australia

We are passionate about exploring the pioneering field of Emotional Intelligence and Heart Intelligence. The heart and breath link our body, mind, emotions and soul. Heart Intelligence is about living a life with connection at all these levels.

Australian Institute of Self Development
http://www.selfdevelopment.com.au/
Ph: 03 9722 2678   Wonga Park, Victoria

Combining EFT, NLP and Time Line Therapy into a unique, super powerful performance coaching framework, The Australian Institute of Self Development has helped thousands of Australians live a life of passion, power and purpose.

USA

HeartMath
http://www.heartmath.com/   California, USA
Ph: 1800 450 9111

HeartMath LLC is an internationally recognised company dedicated to facilitating heart-based living – people relying on the intelligence of their heart in concert with their minds to improve health, performance, relationships and well-being at home and in the workplace.

We have been educating people about stress and emotional management for more than a decade and offer practical, easy-to-use techniques, processes and technology needed for living rewarding, healthy and productive lives.

Alternative Medicine Foundation
http://www.amfoundation.org/   Pontomac, Maryland, USA
Ph: 301-340-1960 (VM only)

Go To Information / General Topics / Find a Practitioner.
Go To Information / Modalities / Acupuncture, Ayurveda, Herbal Medicine, Tibetan Medicine and much more.

The Alternative Medicine Foundation is a non profit organisation, founded in March 1998 to provide responsible and reliable information about alternative medicine to the public and health professionals.

Chapter 13: *Resource Directory*

BUDDHISM & MINDFULNESS

His Holiness the Dalai Lama in Australia
http://www.dalailamainaustralia.org/   Paddington, NSW
Ph: 02 9575 4888
Go To "Buddhist Centres" a list of those around Australia.

December 2009 visit. Our Future, Who is Responsible?
1-10th Dec, Sydney, Hobart, Melbourne.

Mindfulness
http://www.mindfulness.org.au/   Carlton, Victoria
Go To "Links"   for an extensive list of worldwide Mindfulness
            organisations.
Go To "Links / Finding Mindfulness classes" for classes anywhere in
            the world.
Ph: 03 9347 4300

Dr Chris Walsh MBBS, DPM, FAChAM is a psychiatrist working in
private practice in North Carlton (Melbourne, Australia). He has
been working in psychiatry since 1985. In that time, he has worked in
hospitals, jails, community settings, and drug and alcohol institutions.
In 1983, as a young doctor Chris did a short stint helping out at the
Tibetan refugee hospital in Dharamsala. The Tibetan people's common
sense, good humour and happy nature left a lasting impression on him.
Chris's daily mindfulness practice began eighteen months later, at the
same time as he began working in psychiatry. As a result mindfulness
has been organically integrated into his psychiatric practice from the
very start.

USA

Mind and Life Institute
http://www.mindandlife.org/index.html   Boulder, CO
Ph: 303 530 1940

Vision: To establish mutually respectful working collaboration and
research partnerships between modern science and Buddhism — two
of the world's most fruitful traditions for understanding the nature of
reality and promoting human well-being.

"With the ever growing impact of science on our lives, religion and
spirituality have a greater role to play reminding us of our humanity.
There is no contradiction between the two. Each gives us valuable
insights into the other. Both science and the teachings of the Buddha
tell us of the fundamental unity of all things."
The Dalai Lama

INDIA

His Holiness The 14th Dalai Lama of Tibet
http://www.dalailama.com/   Dharamsala, India

For Latest News, Teachings, Webcasts, Messages & Speeches and A Routine Day of HH The Dalai Lama.

About the Author

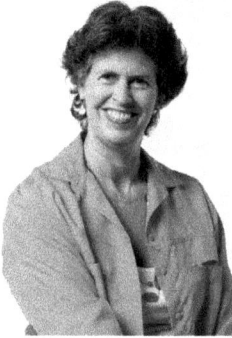

Tracey Stranger has a Bachelor of Applied Science (Microbiology), Graduate Diploma of Marketing, has Certificates in Time Line Therapy, Rebirth Practitioner, Gnana Yoga Meditation, Self Healing & Leadership and is a Natural Health Writer.

Born in Melbourne and curious from a young age her favourite show was Prof Julius Sumner Miller – Why Is It So? Curious to understand how the body works, Tracey studied Microbiology then Business Marketing, working in Sales, Marketing, Business Development and Management at leading Melbourne Hospitals and Pharmaceutical companies.

At the same time Tracey was seeking deeper meaning and understanding at personal development, natural healing, yoga and meditation workshops. Tracey has since taught Taoist Self Healing and Meditation throughout Melbourne and Queensland and guided many to connect deeper within themselves to find meaning and passion. Add fire-walking (without getting burnt feet!), paragliding, husky dog sledding in Greenland to name a few, showing mind over matter and dreams can all come true!

Curious to "learn what happens on the other side of the world", Tracey travelled extensively overseas and learnt "We are all just the same – everyone wants love and connection", plus there is the magnificent variety and spice of life with different cultures.

Returning to Australia and moving to Queensland, Tracey began Consulting in the Natural Health Industry, researching published scientific articles on herbal medicines, ensuring quality manufacturing, laboratory testing and clinical effectiveness. As elected President of Queensland Nutraceutical Industry Association (not-for-profit) for over 7 years, Tracey represented the natural health industry nationally and internationally at Conferences and Austrade events. With truth, quality and integrity Tracey has helped countless individuals in Australia and overseas, personally and in business. Knowing where to go for information and advice, having someone who will listen and understand difficulties, Tracey knows there is always a solution, there can be a win-win, believing adversity and chaos are necessary to drive us toward clarity and harmony.

In 2006, Tracey bought Essential Health Australia Pty Ltd: essential oils to nourish and nurture body and soul. Meditation is a daily routine, discipline bringing freedom, an ever growing sense of self and stronger intuition. The power of meditation and the breath are enormous. Being grateful and saying Yes to life opens the door to endless possibilities.

Travelling and living between Melbourne and Queensland, Tracey's personal interests are in the Ancient Wisdom Teachings and the magic of Meditation. Her passion continues to be to learn and grow and share to help others.

The human body is truly incredible with the ability to heal itself, when we stop putting in toxins (food and thoughts) and nourish (food and thought) ourselves. Tracey is passionate about helping people be the best they can be in health, wealth and happiness, for the good of humanity and the good of our planet and its resources.

www.ingramcontent.com/pod-product-compliance
Lightning Source LLC
Chambersburg PA
CBHW072222270326
41930CB00010B/1956